TRAIL MAP TO
MUSCLE

This book is dedicated to my fiance Sarah

Health Disclaimer

The information and products described in this book have not been evaluated by the Food and Drug Administration and are not intended to diagnose, treat, cure, or prevent any disease or medical conditions. The information in this book and websites reference in this book are not intended as medical advice and should not substitute advice from a healthcare professional. Please consult with your physician or other healthcare provider if you have health related questions before using any of the products or relying on any information you obtain from this book or related websites You should discuss any medications or nutritional supplements you are using with a healthcare provider before using any new medications or supplements.

Always review the labels, warnings, and directions included with any supplement or product before using or consuming the product and do not rely solely on the information in this book or websites recommended in this book.

ISBN: 978-1-7347079-0-8 (print)

ISBN: 978-1-7347079-1-5(ebook)

Ordering Information:

Special discounts are available on quantity purchases by corporations,

associations, and others. For details, contact:

Trailmaptomuscle@gmail.com

www.trailmaptomuscle.com

CONTENTS

TRAIL MAP TO MUSCLE

HOW TO DEFEAT GENETICS, DISEASE, AND BUILD A CONFIDENT BODY

JEREMY MOORE

MY STORY

Growing up, I was always the small, skinny kid among my classmates and friends. I longed to be bigger, put on muscle, and develop strength and watched as others physically matured faster than me. I wondered why I seemed so different, but it was not until age 15, and a year of misdiagnoses, that I discovered the reason: I had cystic fibrosis.

Even though I had the disease since birth, none of its usual symptoms had appeared. Cystic fibrosis (CF) is an inherited disease that causes severe damage to the lungs, digestive system, and other organs, impairing nutrition absorption and healthy growth. However, through the use of digestive enzymes and daily breathing treatments, I was able to slowly put on weight and become healthier.

Even though my cardiovascular activity is limited, I developed the strong body and muscle I have today using the techniques in this book. Just think: if these methods worked for me with my physical challenges, imagine what they can do for you.

I spent many years comparing myself to others every time I walked into a gym. I compared their workouts, form, muscle size, and definition to mine. Even if they weighed more than me and were taller than me, I still would compare myself to them. What was I doing wrong? I thought. What were they doing right? I saw that they were doing the same exercises as me, and sometimes even using lighter weights, but they still had bigger muscles! This drove me crazy until I realized that no other body is like yours.

We're unique, and the ways we process food, our genetics, workouts, and experience all factor into the outcome. Some people just naturally put on muscle or gain strength with ease. The truth is that you can try to improve only one body, and care about one body, and that is your own.

You are your only competition.

You may relate now to how I felt when I began my strength-building journey. I didn't know which exercises to do, how to do them, or the number of sets and reps to include. I had no idea how to use exercise machines or how to perform even a simple bench press. When I tried to organize what little knowledge I had, it all seemed confusing. Every online article, magazine, or book I found on the subject of weightlifting appeared to provide conflicting information. I didn't know where to turn to get results.

Fifteen years later, including 10 years spent as a certified personal trainer, I know how to navigate the path to building the body you desire. I've been in your shoes and understand if some obstacles are making it extra hard for you to start lifting weights and putting on muscle. I'm also ready to guide those of you who have already been working out but want to learn more and discover better ways of moving forward. I'm here to serve as your trail guide.

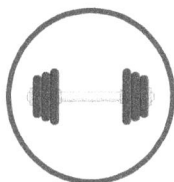

PART 1:
GETTING TRAIL READY

CHAPTER 1

BEGINNING YOUR JOURNEY

"Do something today that your
future self will thank you for."
~ Sean Patrick Flanery, actor, author, and martial artist

Putting in hundreds, even thousands of hours, in the gym over your lifetime to achieve your dream physique takes determination and persistence. It requires countless days when you don't feel like going to the gym. Above all else, you also need to know how to achieve your goal.

Without goals and a roadmap to your destination, you'll waste a lot of time and energy. In this book, I'll help you figure out what you want and how to achieve it.

An excellent place to start is by asking yourself these four questions:

1. Why do I want to change my body?
2. What motivates me to want to lift weights or build on the weightlifting I'm already doing?
3. Am I willing to put in the time and learn about what I need to achieve my goals?
4. Am I willing to put in the work in the gym to achieve my desired physique?

Write down your answers, keep them someplace safe, and refer back to them in the future. When you are not feeling motivated to work out, review them as a reminder of why you started on your journey in the first place.

You may be thinking, what if I'm a beginner?

Anyone can begin lifting weights and exercising, at any age. You may have had an injury or illness, spent decades being sedentary, or just suddenly decided it's time to get in shape. When it comes to beginner weightlifting, I define a beginner as someone who has never lifted weights or has done only push-ups and sit-ups. This book provides you with every bit of information you need to have at this early stage before you advance to intermediate and advanced weightlifting.

Beginner Benchmarks

You can hope to achieve a few goals as a beginner, such as being able to do 10 push-ups, hold a 30-second plank, and perform a pull-up. As you progress, you'll have benchmarks related to lifting weights, such as being able to bench press anywhere from 135 to 315 pounds as well as squatting and deadlifting those same weights.

The transition from beginner to intermediate is marked by building a decent amount of muscle, adding more complicated lifts, combined with the consistent habits of 6 to 12 months of training. Moving from intermediate to advanced lifting typically comes after the two-year mark, when training increases to seven days a week with a greater focus on advanced isolation exercises.

Winning from the Beginning

Many people get excited when beginning a new workout routine, especially at the start of a new year, but most don't continue. I believe the reason for this isn't a lack of motivation but a lack of knowledge. In fact, according to LifeHack.org, 90 percent of people stop exercising after only three months of going to the gym. By following the trail map laid out in this book, you will not be one of these people.

CHAPTER 2

MAPPING THE TERRAIN

"If you can't measure it, you can't improve it."
~ Peter Drucker, educator and author

Before starting your new workout plan, you need to assess where you are now. The goal here is to find your starting point, which serves as the first marker on the path to your desired destination or goal.

Measurements, fitness testing, and photographs will give you the most accurate overview of your body. The first thing I suggest is taking your photo and then completing your measurements. You'll want to save the fitness testing portion for last because the blood in your muscles will affect your body measurements. Doing these assessments monthly provides you with specific feedback on your progress. It gives you an idea of which muscles are developing and which ones are lagging behind and, in doing so, serves as a motivational tool.

Photo

For the photo, set the timer on your phone camera or have someone take a picture of you in the least amount of clothing you feel comfortable wearing so that you can see as much of your body as possible. Take a full head-to-toe frontal body photo, a head-to-toe side profile, a head-to-toe back photo, and photos from the front and back while performing a double flexed biceps pose.

A double-flexed biceps pose requires holding your arms up in the traditional strongman pose and contracting your biceps as tight as possible. Make sure the lighting is adequate so that nothing appears shaded. Keep these photos in a safe and convenient place because you'll want to refer back to them on a monthly or quarterly basis. You may want to retake them at some point for side-by-side comparisons.

If you retake the photos later, try to match the previous conditions before working out and wear the same clothes. For measurements, find a tailor's measuring tape or order a Gulick or MyoTape tape measure online.

Measuring Tapes

Gulick measuring tapes are the most accurate and consistent way to take measurements. They have a pull pin with a marker line that allows for the same tension on each reading. MyoTapes allow for easy at-home measurements because the end of the tape attaches to the device and uses spring tension to provide accuracy. The MyoTape works best if you intend to do the measurements yourself. If not, you'll want to have someone help you take the following measurements: biceps, shoulders, chest, waist, abdominals, hips, thighs, and calves, in no particular order.

Here are some helpful tips on how to take each measurement:

Biceps: Wrap tape around middle point or peak of the bicep, flexed and unflexed.

Shoulders: With both arms down at your side, wrap tape at the middle of the shoulder line around the body.

Chest: Wrap tape around the body across the nipple line, measuring just the torso, arms at your side. Put tape under both arms, being careful not to include the arms in the measurement.

Abdominals: Tape goes around the torso approximately one inch above the belly button.

Waist: Tape should be across the belly button all the way around the body.

Hips: Tape is around your hips at the point where the glutes (buttocks) are widest.

Thighs: Take measurements for each leg with the tape around each quad at the widest part of the leg, above the knee but below the hips.

Calves: Take measurement for each calf with the tape around the widest point of the calf muscle.

After recording all of your measurements, it's time to assess your basic strength levels. An excellent place to start is with a push-up test.

Strength Assessment

Find an object that is about three inches high, such as a yoga block laid flat or a couple of stacked books. Make a note of what you use so that future tests for comparison are the same. Perform as many push-ups as you can, touching your chest to the object each time. There's no time limit and the only resting period is at the top of the movement. For proper form, keep your elbows slightly tucked in by your torso, keeping the head looking towards the floor. Keep your entire body flat and don't let your hips sag towards the floor. If you can't perform regular push-ups on your toes, try them on your knees instead, and be sure to note the type you did.

Next, perform a plank. To achieve a proper plank, start with your knees off the ground in a push-up position, then drop down onto your forearms and elbows, keeping the rest of the body straight. Make sure your body is parallel to the ground, holding the back of the head in line with your spine. You can also use a mirror placed on the ground if you want to assess your form.

Make sure your belly button is pulled in and squeeze the buttocks as tight as possible.

Breathe normally, even though it may become more difficult the longer you hold this position. If you feel most of your weight on the elbows and shoulders, your core isn't doing the work. Record your time. Now let's move one step closer towards your first workout.

CHAPTER 3

PREPARING WITH THE BASICS

If you've ever been in a gym or talked to someone about lifting weights, you have probably heard words such as sets, reps, dumbbells, or barbells. These and many more terms that make up the lingo of weightlifting must be understood to begin building a muscular body.

Here are the essential terms:

Barbell: A long metal bar measuring four to seven feet long that allows for additional weight plates to be placed on each end. A barbell falls into the category of free weights. It's the bar used to hold the most weight and is mostly used on compound exercises such as the squat, deadlift, military press, and bench press.

Compound movement: A multi-joint movement and a lift that builds the most muscle and recruits multiple muscle groups. Examples include squats and bench press.

Concentric: The lifting phase of a movement, shortening the muscle as it acts against resistance. An example of the concentric portion of a lift would be curling a dumbbell from your waist up to your shoulder.

Dumbbell: A fixed weight attached to a short handle. Also, in the free weights family, dumbbells allow for individual movements such as curls, shoulder presses, and dumbbell chest presses. Dumbbells range in weight from 1 pound to more than 150 pounds.

Eccentric: The return phase of a movement, slowing the motion that lengthens muscles while producing force. An example of an eccentric portion of a lift would be the lowering of a dumbbell from the shoulder to the hips.

Forced rep: A rep (one complete exercise motion) performed with a spotter, who helps you go past where you would stop on your own. An example would be a spotter helping to take a bit of the weight off of a lift so you can get through the hardest part of a movement and do a few more reps. Forced reps are typically only for intermediate or advanced lifters.

Free weight: A type of weight unattached to a machine. Free weights, which include dumbbells and barbells, are used in most strength training exercises. They're important for many reasons, such as recruiting stabilizer muscles and allowing the body to move in its most natural pattern.

Failure: When you've completed a movement to the point where the intended muscle is depleted and can't perform another rep. It's usually saved for the last set of a muscle group and is an advanced training principle.

Hypertrophy: Muscle growth due to tearing down muscle fibers, then rebuilding them to make them stronger.

Isolation movement: A single joint exercise that focuses on one muscle group at a time— for instance, dumbbell curls.

Plate: A hard rubber or metal disc ranging in weight from about 2 pounds to 45 pounds. The standard weights for most big lifts call for at least one 45-pound plate on each side of the bar.

Primary muscles: Muscles that are the most in control of any movement. In other words, they're the targeted muscles during an exercise.

Rep: One complete motion of an exercise. Reps are important for many reasons including the fact that knowing the number of reps determines the amount of weight to be used.

Set: A group of consecutive repetitions. Determining how many sets of an exercise you will perform can be critical to your workout and long-term success. Too few or too many sets can each have their downfalls. Choosing whether to do a set with one piece of equipment over another is also important.

Secondary muscles: Muscles that assist the targeted muscles in completing an exercise, sometimes taking over when the primary muscle fails.

Spotter: Someone who assists with an exercise if the motion can't be completed or needs slight assistance to complete it safely.

Superset: Performing two exercises back to back of different body parts.

Training split: Focusing on different muscle groups on separate days. For instance, you could do back and biceps on Monday, then chest and triceps on Tuesday.

One rep max: The most amount of weight you can lift during an exercise for one rep.

While many more phrases and terms are addressed later in the book, these terms provide a foundation for your training and are the most vital to know as you start out.

CHAPTER 4

UNDERSTANDING MUSCLES

Before we begin learning exercises and how to train each body part, let's break down each muscle group and understand the various parts. It's essential to study and understand muscles you use or should use for a particular lift. Let's take a look at muscles, breaking them down into large and small muscle groups, to better understand their makeup and function.

LARGE MUSCLE GROUPS

Chest muscles

The chest, which is the most over-trained muscle (because it's what everyone looks at!), includes pectoralis major and pectoralis minor muscles. The pectoralis major, or pecs, make up the majority of the chest muscles. The chest is primarily trained using heavy presses such as incline, flat, and decline bench presses as well as push-ups. You use the pec minor during exercises such as chest flyes and dips.

Back muscles

Back muscles consist of the latissimus dorsi, teres major, trapezius, erector spinae, and rhomboids. Building a strong back is important for many aspects of daily life, from improving your posture to helping you carry groceries. However, it comes in second to legs when men undertrain. Since you can't see back muscles easily, workouts tend to lean towards less intensity and shorter duration. Some of the essential exercises for building a strong back are deadlifts, pull-ups, and rows.

Leg muscles

Leg muscles include quads, hamstrings, and glutes. Of the three muscle groups, legs have most growth potential because of the amount of muscle you can target in one workout. Still, legs are undertrained in men because they will get stronger but may not grow as fast as the chest or biceps. Common leg exercises include squats, lunges, step-ups, and leg press.

SMALL MUSCLE GROUPS

Deltoids

Deltoids, or delts, are the shoulder muscles and include the anterior, middle, and posterior deltoids. Male weightlifters favor these muscles because they're so visible. The delts have three parts: the front, middle, and rear, the latter being the least trained to the extent that is needed.

Triceps

Triceps include two-thirds of the arm and are essential for building arm size. They also assist the chest in exercises like dips and bench presses. The bigger your triceps, the bigger your arms will look overall. The triceps have three heads: The lateral, long, and medial head. To achieve what is called the "horseshoe" shape of the triceps, it's necessary to concentrate on all three to develop size, strength, and symmetry. Exercises for building bigger triceps include close and reverse grip bench press, dips, and overhead dumbbell triceps extensions.

Biceps

Biceps are composed of two heads—the short and long heads. Working the biceps won't put a lot of size on your arm or frame in general, but they're a critical part of having a balanced physique. Popular biceps exercises include dumbbell curls and chin-ups.

Trapezius

The trapezius, or traps, are located in the upper body and run from the middle of the upper back up into the neck. The traps are essential for building a great physique. Exercises such as shrugs, upright rows, pull-ups, and farmer walks all build the traps well.

Abdominals

The abdominals, or abs, are one of the primary aesthetic muscles desired by most men. They include the interior and exterior oblique, erectus abdominis, transverse and rectus abdominis. If a man has visible abs, it means his body fat is below 10 percent.

Calves

The calves are the muscles most neglected by men. Genetics play a significant factor in their growth and natural size. They include the soleus and gastrocnemius, and their main building exercises are seated and standing calf raises.

Muscle Group Training

When you're trying to build the most muscle, you must primarily train the three large muscle groups. The smaller groups can have their own training day or you can add them onto the end of a large muscle group workout. While important, they won't provide the growth that comes from big large muscle lifts. When beginning your journey, you'll see significant improvements in strength and growth from the large muscle groups then subsequent growth from the smaller groups that assist in bigger lifts.

For example, when you're doing a bench press, shoulders and triceps are doing much of the work to help control weight on the concentric (pressing away) as well as eccentric (lowering bar back to chest) parts of the lift. Equally, during a pull-up, the biceps help make the exercise more manageable. The abs also come into play on an exercise such as a pull-up or chin-up and will strengthen accordingly.

Understanding your body's muscles will allow you to truly understand the ones that are activated in each exercise you perform. It will also help you develop an idea of the exact groups that are lagging behind in your training program.

Before we get into how to perform exercises, let's first consider where you will be lifting weights.

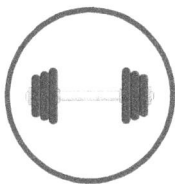

PART 2:
CHOOSING YOUR ADVENTURE

CHAPTER 5

WORKING OUT AT HOME

Deciding where you will work out is one of the most critical elements to consider before attempting to build muscle and get in shape. Ask yourself these questions: What is the best option financially? Which location is most convenient? What will give you the best results in the least amount of time?

A home gym is a very appealing option for many reasons. If you have time constraints and want to make sure you do your workout, a home gym could be your best option. It's also a good option if you have a limited budget, don't have easy access to transportation, or have an open garage or spare room for equipment. Whether you start with a pair of push-up handles or a doorway pull-up bar, having a home gym can be a big step towards making progress toward your goals.

Some common home gym items include dumbbells, a door mounted pull up bar, and a bench press with a leg extension attached at the end. Though this bare-bones equipment will get you some progress, it doesn't scratch the surface of what you need to be serious about putting on muscle.

Choosing to build and work out in a home gym has its advantages. You don't have to leave the house and drive to a gym and sit in traffic, only to get there and have to wait to use your desired equipment. You can buy the exact equipment you want, and you don't have to worry about someone else sweating all over it and not cleaning it. There are also no outside distractions at a home gym, such as other people talking to you or being distracted by watching others. With a home gym, you also have privacy to work out in any outfit—without judgment.

Deciding to use a home gym has its drawbacks as well. First, you may be limited by space for equipment and exercises. I recommend measuring the space to ensure equipment will fit, especially since it can be expensive. Another disadvantage is that you're alone and it's much harder to motivate yourself. To remedy this, I suggest cutting out some fitness magazine photos with your desired body type and placing them around the gym.

Choosing the Right Equipment

To best equip your home gym, let's take a look at commonly used equipment to learn what you'll need and how to maximize its use.

Dumbbells

Men who start to lift weights at home often buy a spin-lock dumbbell bar kit. The kit includes a dumbbell with threads at each end that allows for small weight plates to be screwed onto them. Most of these kits come with weight plates totaling up to about 20 pounds per dumbbell with combinations of 2.5-pound to 10-pound plates. The major disadvantage of using these dumbbells is that you will spend more time constantly screwing and unscrewing the different plates to get your desired weight. They also don't allow for supersets, giant sets, pyramids, or any other training principle which involves using different amounts of weights back to back.

A better option, though more expensive, is to purchase dumbbells such as the Bowflex SelectTech series. Each dumbbell allows for quick change-outs from 2.5 pounds to 52.5 pounds. If you're committed to training at home, these are a great way to train many body parts.

Bench press rack

The bench press rack is a must-have in any gym, especially a home gym. A home-grade quality bench can vary in price from $70 to over $500. Make sure it's sturdy, wide enough for your frame, and that you have a stable surface on which to place it. If there is any wobble or potential of collapse, you won't be able to perform your set confidently and perhaps risk injury.

You'll need a separate bench for other exercises such as incline curls, decline dumbbell chest presses, incline dumbbell chest presses, and rows, among others. Make sure both benches can decline as well as incline, which will allow you to get much more use out of your home gym setup. For the bench press, you'll also have to purchase an Olympic bar and weight plates ranging from 5-45 pounds.

Pull-up and chin-up equipment

This equipment can be as simple as a doorway or freestanding pull-up bar. If you purchase a door mount pull-up bar, be sure that it has multiple grips, which will allow for more exercises than just regular pull-ups and chin-ups. Secure it into the doorway or hook it onto the top of the molding so that you can trust it won't break loose and injure you. If you purchase the freestanding option, it will have a pull-up bar attached to a frame that includes a back pad for ab knee raises and two handles for dips, all in one piece of equipment. This option is more stable and safer than any doorway pull-up bar.

Squat racks

There are two types of squat racks found in most home gyms. One is a simple rack that holds the bar at a pre-adjusted height between two poles with a small cradle at the top to rest the bar. The other is a power rack which features adjustable hooks and safety rails in case you are unable to finish the squat. The bar and weights you use for your bench press can be used in either type of squat rack, so you will not have to purchase a second set. Having the proper equipment for squats will allow you to do exercises that add mass to your lower body.

Small and portable equipment

If your home gym space is limited in size, there are equipment options such as wall-mounted squat racks that fold up and store out of the way. Also, some benches have wheels that allow for them to be moved easily to the side of your home gym space, if needed. If you plan to purchase any cardio equipment, including an exercise bike or elliptical, check to see how easily they can be moved so you can use the space when you aren't working out.

Where to purchase home equipment

For a basic home setup, my best suggestion is to purchase new less expensive items, such as a door-mounted pull-up bar, and find the rest used on Craigslist or an app such as Offer Up. You can often find almost-new equipment at half the cost, and it may not have much wear and tear. Be sure to check reviews on any items you order online to confirm it is top quality and will fit your fitness needs.

Equipment can start to add up, so make sure it will last. Remember that for the price of about half of this equipment (new or used), you can afford a gym membership for many years. Home gyms can be great with the right equipment, but don't expect to get the same results you would from a regular gym or health club.

The diversity of equipment at most gyms is hard to match in a home setup.

Equipment upgrades

Before you start, assess your current equipment and if you need to or are able to make small upgrades. This can be in the form of buying more dumbbells, a long bar, workout bench, or a door mounted pull-up bar. I recommend at least having interchangeable dumbbells. They aren't optimal but do allow for many different dumbbell weights without having to buy a full set. If nothing else, you can use a milk jug filled all or halfway with water as long as it's the kind with a secure screw-on cap.

Also, a quality door-mounted pull-up bar is essential to working on your back. I also suggest purchasing exercise bands, which are rubber tubes attached to two handles. Bands are relatively inexpensive and can be attached to a doorway and used for many exercises, at various heights and angles. Bands also can provide a lot of resistance with the tubing not taking up much room. If you're using the door attachment, be sure to lock the door so someone doesn't open the door and injure you.

At-home cardio

For cardio at home, many options, such as using a local school track, cost nothing. If you live at the beach, you can run or walk in the sand. Bike riding and skateboarding are also good cheap cardio options.

Having a treadmill, elliptical, or exercise bike at home is great but can have drawbacks. Sometimes having the equipment in your house can make it less desirable to use and easier to stop working out earlier than you should. Also, what started out as a good intention can slowly turn into a place to hang clothes. If you enjoy running, or want to start running, I suggest visiting your local running store to make sure you have proper athletic shoes and avoid injuring yourself. I tried to run when I was beginning my fitness journey and wasn't able to finish a mile because of the pain in my feet from not having shoes that fit well. A running store can provide you with the right shoe based on your natural foot movement when you walk and run.

I don't recommend a lot of cardio if you're trying primarily to build muscle mass. But if your first main goal is to shed body fat, add more cardio to your routine with somewhere between three to four sessions a week. (See Chapter 26 for more details.)

If you do decide to work out at home, all of the workouts in this book can be modified to fit your equipment. This might take a little creativity but it's achievable. You can do many barbell exercises with dumbbells instead, and you can substitute lat pulldowns by using the pull-up assist band I mentioned earlier.

CHAPTER 6

GOING TO A GYM

Walking into a gym on the first day can seem overwhelming. The vast amount of equipment to choose from and the number of other people working out can be intimidating. It helps to first make sure a gym is right for you.

Let's take a look at why joining a gym can be a superior choice over working out at home gym and then discuss choosing the type of gym that works best for your desired physique.

Pros and Cons

A gym with quality machines, a full range of dumbbells, as well as all of the weight plates you need for any exercise makes it a breeze to move through a planned workout. But it can also be a potential danger to someone who doesn't know which machines to use or how to use them properly. (See Chapter 17 for more details.)

The gym also can be a great place to learn new exercises and techniques by watching others who are more experienced than you. For instance, you may see someone use a machine in a new way and add that particular exercise to your routine.

Most gyms will have more equipment than one could ever

have at home, though that might mean having to wait. There's nothing more frustrating than having a preplanned workout routine and showing up to the gym only to have all of the squat racks, cable stations, and pull-up bars taken. Knowing how to work around this and being able to modify your routine on the fly comes with time.

A key to avoiding this issue is to work out during off-peak times that don't correspond with the average person's nine-to-five work schedule. Mondays at most gyms are typically very busy in the afternoon and evening. Monday is also "International Chest Day," so expect all of the benches to be in use during peak times. Because of this, it's an excellent time to start your week with your weakest body part. For most guys, this is either their legs or back. Mondays are also typically the day most guys hit the gym the hardest, so training your weakest body part will give it what it needs to grow and catch up.

Choosing a Gym

The first factor to consider when joining a gym is the location. How far do you live from local gyms, and how do you determine which type is the best fit for you? The first question is critical. Typically, you want to find a gym that is 5–15 minutes from your home or workplace. Anything farther away than that can lead to skipped workouts. You may need to travel a little farther if none of the nearby gyms match your intended training style.

Starting your regimen at a gym designed for the general public may be the best option. Some gyms are tailored towards men who have already been lifting for quite some time and have specific goals, such as strength or bodybuilding.

You'll recognize mainstream gyms, which include local recreational centers, by their dumbbells maxing out at 100 pounds, pop music playing over the speakers, and an equal balance of men and women working out. Most rec centers are a low-cost option with fees as low as $75 for the year, versus big box gyms that charge $45 a month or more and require a yearly contract.

Many 24-hour gym chains are a decent option. They have costs as low as $10 a month and no long-term commitment. Alternatively, some gyms require an upfront payment and then charge the monthly rate.

CHAPTER 7

SCHEDULING YOUR WORKOUTS

Maximizing your workouts and your training time means finding the best exercise schedule. Three days a week is all you'll need to start building muscle and noticing changes and scheduling your week and workouts ahead of time is vital.

Training the same muscle groups twice a week can be done but only if those muscles have fully recovered. On average, give a muscle group at least 48–72 hours to recover and rebuild before working out again. You'll notice that specific muscles recover quicker than others, and as you progress in training over weeks and months, most muscles will recover faster and faster depending upon the intensity of the workout. You may need to do some workouts in the morning, midday, or evening.

Ask yourself: When is the best time for me to work out? How will I know which body parts to work out and when?

Timing Your Workouts

Early Morning. Some people work out in the early morning because of their work schedule. One good thing about working out earlier in the day is that your workout will be done and out of the way. You have to prioritize your workout over other things in your life if you want to make the best gains possible. Let me repeat that because it's of the utmost importance: *You have to prioritize your workout over other things in your life if you want to make the best possible gains!* The only way to do this is by sticking to a schedule and maintaining consistency.

Midday. The middle of the day at a gym is usually the least busy time and a great time to do your lifts. If you have this option, even for one day out of the week, take advantage of it. More than likely, the equipment you want to use will be available and you'll have more room in which to perform your exercises.

Evening. I don't suggest training in the evening if you don't have to. If you work out after work, there's always a chance of being too tired or not having the motivation to do the workout. Working out late can sometimes make it hard to fall asleep and your energy from the day may be almost completely used up. The gym is typically busier in the evening and you may get frustrated when even the secondary equipment is taken.

When to Train Different Parts of the Body

You may be wondering when each body part should be trained. The day and muscles you train is called a "split." A split depends on your available days to train, weaker versus stronger body parts, and which phase you are in. If you're just starting out, I suggest giving each body part its own day. A sample week would look like the following:

Monday: Legs
Tuesday: Chest
Wednesday: Back
Thursday: Triceps
Friday: Shoulders
Saturday: Biceps
Sunday: Abs

A typical split week should begin with your weakest body part. The next day should be a muscle that is not impacted by the previous day. An example would be to do chest training on Monday and biceps or back on Tuesday. After the first few weeks of training, you can begin to superset body parts on certain days. An example of that split would be:

Monday: Legs
Tuesday: Chest and Back
Wednesday: Rest or Abs
Thursday: Biceps and Triceps
Friday: Rest
Saturday: Shoulders and Abs
Sunday: Rest

Deciding on the best split for you will take some experimentation, and your splits may change along your journey. Feel free to arrange your rest days and when you choose to do your ab training.

Sometimes when you don't feel like getting to the gym and instead want to stay home and postpone it until the next day, a strategy that works well is just getting yourself *to* the gym. Once you're there, you'll see others working out and become motivated. Even if you tell yourself that you are just going to go for 15 minutes, 15 will turn into 30, and 30 will turn into an hour.

If you're still having trouble with motivation, pull out your first day photos and reasons for starting your journey, or turn to Chapter 1 of this book and reread it. *Just do something. Anything is better than nothing.* If you work out at home, ask yourself, "What point in the day will I have the most energy?" Some men find that getting a hard workout in the morning revs them up and clears their head for the day. On the other hand, working out in the evening may be the best option because you can burn off stress from the day and turn it into motivation to work out much harder.

One other way to make yourself work harder and get better results during your workouts is to find a workout partner.

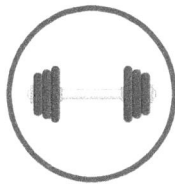

PART 3:
KNOW BEFORE YOU GO

CHAPTER 8
FINDING A TRAIL BUDDY

There's nothing wrong with going it alone in pursuit of your dream physique. However, having a workout partner can accelerate your gains and keep you accountable for doing your workouts. Finding a gym partner that is more or less at your same level of fitness is the hard part.

One way to find a workout partner is to look for others who typically work out around the same time as you do and tend to lift roughly the same weight. Introduce yourself by asking him to spot you or asking if he needs a spot, which can spark a conversation and lead to a consistent workout partner. If you can't find someone at your same level, you may find someone who is in better shape than you. That can be advantageous, helping you work your way up to the weights your partner uses. The disadvantage is that it can become tedious during a workout to continually change out weights for compound exercises, such as bench press and squats.

Pros of Having a Partner

Overall, gym partners have many benefits. When you aren't feeling motivated to work out, they can push you through. Also, you know they're already on their way to the gym to meet you or are there waiting for you. During your workout, you have someone to talk to, exchange workout and exercise advice, and most important, someone there to spot you. If they're at your same experience level, you'll learn and make mistakes together and celebrate gains as well.

They can also push you to do more weight than you think you are capable of doing. Just having them there to spot you can take the worry away about dropping the weight or not being able to finish the lift. That confidence can push you to new strength levels. Workouts become more fun and safer since they can help correct your form. There can also be a certain amount of competition to keep you pushing harder. The more comfortable you are with each other, the more likely you are to call each other out for being lazy or not pushing yourself to the max.

Cons of Having a Partner

Difficulties involve what to do when your workout buddy can't make it to the gym himself. Make sure the person you choose is dependable, trustworthy, and ready to dedicate themselves to your routine. You also can always have more than one workout partner. If for some reason your main partner can't make it, you can call the other person and ask if they would like to do the workout you've planned.

If your schedules start to clash, it may be time to find another partner. If you see that your workout partner talks a lot or find yourself talking a lot during your workouts, it may be time to have an honest conversation about what you can both do to improve your workout as a whole. Too much conversation can mean you can go minutes between sets and slowly lose the momentum you had at the start.

CHAPTER 9

TRAIL TUNES

Almost everyone I meet who lifts weights alone listens to music when they're working out at a gym or at home. Music provides a push and increased focus, and it can make a massive difference in the intensity of your workout. Most gyms play music but it's usually not loud enough or sufficiently upbeat enough to push you to work harder. My best suggestion is to bring your own music and headphones.

If you're playing music from your phone, be sure to have enough music available on it to create a playlist. You may also choose to use a streaming service's playlist such as Pandora or Spotify. Creating or deciding on a playlist for the workout ahead of time can get you pumped up. Selecting a specific song order also can help get you through a grueling workout. Set the playlist up beforehand so it doesn't end before the workout is over. If you have to stop to add new songs or restart the playlist, you lose valuable workout time.

Next, how are you going to listen to your music? For me, wireless headphones are a must. Standard headphones can snag or get caught on equipment and rip out of your ears. Having wireless headphones keeps your phone out of your pocket where it won't get smashed by dumbbells resting on your legs. If you choose to use wireless headphones, make sure you charge them before your workout session. If you would rather listen with corded headphones, prevent snagging them on equipment by tucking them inside your shirt, running the cord from your pocket up through the front of your shirt. You can also put your phone in an armband and run the wire through your sleeve and up into your ears with the slack running under your shirt.

When you're listening to music or have a phone in the gym, keep it in your pocket or put it away where you won't be distracted by checking social media or emails. The more time spent away from your set can cause your muscles to get cold. Once muscles get cold, the workout is over. Keep an extra pair of headphones in your vehicle when heading to the gym, even if they're a cheap pair. Nothing is worse than leaving your headphones at home and having to listen to bad music played over gym speakers.

CHAPTER 10

READY TO HIT THE TRAILHEAD

By now, you have a solid foundation of knowledge about your body and training terminology. You've decided where to work out, and you're ready to begin. First, however, you need to know about what to expect if you choose to sign up at a gym and you need to learn about the equipment you'll be using.

Gym Tour

Walking into a gym for the first time can be overwhelming, but there will usually be someone there ready to give you a tour and get you signed up. A good question to ask yourself while touring the facility is, "Will I feel motivated to work out here when I walk through the front door?" Some gyms don't inspire or lack an atmosphere of motivation or energy. Try to do your initial walk-through at the time you intend to use the gym so you can gauge how busy it might be. You should be able to get a feel for what equipment is available as well as its cleanliness and quality.

Signing Up

After the tour, you are typically shown various sign-up options. Some gyms allow for a month-to-month contract but most offer only annual memberships. There is generally an initial sign-up fee but this can be waived by just refusing to pay it and threatening to walk away. Some gyms offer a discount if you pay ahead for the year and they won't need to keep your credit card on file.

Ask about all up-front fees including cancellation charges so you don't find any surprises, like the fees some gyms charge annually to buy new equipment. Find out if a free week pass is available before signing on the dotted line. This pass gives you a chance to give the gym a trial run to determine if it's the best for you. Also, be sure to check with your employer, who may provide gym benefits.

Many people who sign up for gym memberships end up not using them for one reason or another. You're not going to be that person on this journey.

CHAPTER 11

GYM ETIQUETTE

Now that you've chosen a gym and have a good feeling for the layout, it's important to be aware of rules of behavior (some unspoken) so you don't upset other members or lose your membership.

Gym etiquette applies regardless of the gym you choose and apply to everyone.

Clean up. Keeping equipment clean after use is a vital part of gym etiquette. There isn't anything more aggravating than seeing someone sweat all over a bench or machine and then walk away without cleaning it. I once encountered a man walking away from an ab machine covered in sweat. When I confronted him, he replied, "I'm from a real gym." I don't know what that means, but don't be like that guy.

Typically, gyms will provide sanitizing wipes or paper towels with a spray bottle of cleaning solution to wipe down equipment. A safe practice is to wipe down a machine or bench before *and* after use. Sometimes a surface can appear clean that was covered with sweat that's since dried. If you sweat heavily, lay a towel down on the machine while using it and make sure to wipe the sweat off the equipment after use. In addition, be sure to use the provided cleaning solution so you are not just spreading the sweat around.

It's also a good idea to take two towels from the front desk upon entering the gym. Use one to clean machines and one for your face. Don't confuse them! When wiping down equipment after use, make sure to clean the entire surface you touched or that came into contact with your body. Gym members often will quickly wipe down a tiny portion of the equipment so they can say they cleaned it. That's why I suggest pre-wiping down any equipment you use.

Don't work out when sick. In most gyms, you'll find hand sanitizer stations scattered throughout the facility. It's a good idea to use sanitizer two or three times during your workout since many bugs and viruses as well as bacteria spread inside a gym. Always be sure to wash your hands thoroughly before and after every workout because you'll be touching at least 25 different surfaces during your time there. If you aren't feeling well, stay home instead of working out. Not working out is a better choice than the risk of spreading your cold or virus to people within the gym and feeling worse yourself.

Wear clean clothes. Be sure to put on clean clothes for every workout session. You may not realize yourself how bad you smell, especially if you have worn the same shirt for three workouts in a row. Keep a clean shirt, socks, and an extra pair of shorts or pants in your car to grab just in case you forgot them at home.

Properly (and carefully) re-rack weights. A cardinal rule of gym etiquette as crucial as cleanliness is re-racking your weights. Un-racked weights left on the floor can cause injury if someone trips over them or steps on one during an exercise.

Also remember: Re-racking weights is one thing but properly re-racking them is another. Make sure dumbbells are in the appropriate slot for their weight and weight plates are on the corresponding weight pole. Usually gyms have what are called weight trees that can hold multiple 45s, 35s, 25s, 10s, and 5s, as well as dumbbell racks with the designed dumbbell weight printed on the designed slot.

Bench press benches have poles on the back or side with weight numbers for the corresponding poles where the weights belong. Heavier weights typically go on the bottom with the smaller weights on top. You'll also see this configuration on a Smith machine but reversed. The heaviest weights are higher for quicker transitions to the bar for exercises such as squats and lunges.

You'll often find a leg press previously been used by someone who left six plates on each side that have to be completely removed and re-racked for you to use the machine. Typically, at least one 45-pound plate is left on each side of the leg press because most people do at least this amount of weight for their sets. Chances are if someone has left his or her weights on the machine, they probably didn't wipe it down. Someone else may need it after you who can only do a 10-pound weight on each side so it's best to remove all of your weights when you're done.

You'll also usually find bench press stations with the weight left on the bar, either 135 or 225 pounds. Many lifters leave 135 pounds on the bar because it's the weight most generally use for bench press. But if you are warming up, you'll have to remove it. Some gyms have signs that read, "If you are caught leaving weights on the bar, you may have your gym membership suspended." Though I haven't seen this in person, I believe it happens. If someone is consistently not following the rules, other gym-goers will get fed up enough to complain to management.

You may also see a sign that reads, "Do not slam weights." This warning applies to dropping a bar during deadlifts—and even dropping dumbbells. After using dumbbells for an exercise such as chest presses or curls, be sure to lower them to the ground carefully. Don't slam them down because they can hurt you or another gym member. If you need to drop them quickly, it may be a sign that they're too heavy for your sets. You may have heard of this in the form of the lunk alarm (a 110-decibel tornado siren) at Planet Fitness that goes off if weights are slammed.

Don't be a machine hog. Try not to use a machine for more than 10 minutes. Be sure to get right to your set once you get to the equipment, and don't rest for too long.

If someone has your machine next for his or her workout, he or she might come up and stand there hovering, pressuring you to finish and asking, "How many more sets?" You don't want to be that person, making others rush to complete their sets. The proper thing to do is politely get their attention and ask how many sets they have left. If they say they're just getting started, it's best to go ahead and move to another exercise. If they say it's their last set, don't just hover. Simply let it be known to other gym members that you are next in line.

Be courteous. Sometimes you can ask people to leave the weight they're using if it's close to what you'll use. When you're taking over a bench or machine with leftover weights from someone else, you can offer to take them off if there are not too many plates. They'll appreciate the offer. Many times, people waiting to use your machine will clean the machine for you after you are done with your sets.

Frequently, people will leave a towel draped over the equipment or a phone, shaker bottle, or hoodie next to it while they go to grab water or use the restroom. If you see a bench or machine that has nothing around it or on it and you think it's free, you can get the nearest person's attention to ask if it's in use. If they have headphones on, point to the machine and signal to them to nod yes or no. Don't assume equipment is in use just because the weights are still sitting on the bar.

Be mindful. Sometimes you can ask a person using your intended piece of equipment if you can "work-in." Working-in means doing your set in between their working sets while they rest. This is ideal if you are using their same level of weight or close to it. If they're taking a break between sets and the bars are free, you can jump in and use the time they would rest.

You don't want to work-in when you have to take their weight off or break up their routine. If you're working-in for an exercise such as a bench press, be extra sure to lay your towel down on the bench during your sets and remove it immediately after your sets are complete. Sometimes a pair of people working out will ask if they can work-in with you. Politely say "no" because you'll get stuck waiting two minutes or more while they complete their sets.

Get out of the way. A common mistake made by new gym-goers is standing or being in the way of members using the mirror as they perform their exercise. If it appears that you'll be blocking them while you grab dumbbells off a rack, grab your weight quickly and then move out of the way. Also, you don't want to do any exercise while standing right at the dumbbell rack, even if it's just a quick warm-up set. You likewise want to make sure you never get too close to someone doing an exercise such as squats or Olympic lifts. It can be easy to get hit with the end of the bar or have a dropped bar roll onto your foot. Ouch.

Move your gym bag. Most gyms have a no gym bags on the floor policy, though I have actually never seen this enforced. Having a gym bag on the floor is a tripping hazard. I once saw a gym bag left in the main walking area of the dumbbell rack and the owner didn't move it even after seeing others stepping over it.

Put your phone away. Cell phones can be kept near you while you work out if you're using them for music or tracking your workout on an app. It can be easy to be distracted by your phone while working out by sending texts, checking email, or social media between sets. But not only will this take time out of your workout, it will make you "that" cell phone person in the gym.

Limit phone use to time between exercises or turn it to airplane mode so you can't receive any distracting text messages or phone calls. I witnessed the same guy on multiple occasions with a phone held up to his head during his whole workout, from curls to crunches. Talking to someone on the phone for your entire workout through your headphones is bad enough but holding an actual phone is even worse.

Following these rules will help you fit right in at the gym and make your workouts go much smoother. There will always be people who don't heed these rules or don't know any better, but you should never be that person. Learning gym etiquette early on will help you progress faster and keep you on the right track in the gym.

CHAPTER 12

THE ESSENTIAL TENETS OF SUCCESS

Though this is one of the longest chapters in the book, it will be the most important for you to use as a reference now and in the future for maximizing your workout sessions. Let's dive right in.

To achieve your goals, you have to understand and remind yourself where you are heading and why you are doing what you do. That means as you lift heavier and heavier weights and perform more sets with increased intensity, you need to make sure you're continuing to build muscle. Through years of training and research, I've come to understand the fastest and most effective ways of doing this.

Rethink your routine

Many assume that their intended muscle is getting the full benefit of an exercise, but even many of you who have been training for years may need to rethink your routine. Relearning incorrect motor patterns takes time, and it can be challenging to go back to step one and learn the correct way to get the best contraction and results out of each exercise.

Strength through hypertrophy

Building muscle, which is our primary focus, also increases strength. However, because of the law of diminishing returns, muscle growth becomes harder to achieve over time. It means that you start getting less and less out of the same effort and output. Adjusting your routine to continue that growth is of the utmost importance.

New hypertrophy will ignite in a muscle when you learn how to engage specific muscles. For example, if you do a flat bench press and continue to add more and more weight but aren't seeing growth in your chest, it's more than likely because other muscles (such as your shoulders and triceps) are carrying the brunt of the load. In other words, they're getting stronger while your chest remains weak.

Changing your routine and how you do exercises will spark growth, even if you have to go back and start with very light weights to feel the contraction. I recommend starting with your weakest body part and understanding how to contract it throughout every repetition.

Thinking into the Muscle

What does this mean? To think into the muscle simply implies focusing only on the intended muscle and not just going through the exercise motions. The concentration curl is a great example. The word "concentration" is in the name, and this is an exercise that directs your attention to the biceps and feeling every bit of the contraction. This is much more difficult in an exercise such as a lat pulldown, or even a pull-up.

Maintaining this mind-muscle connection keeps you focused on your form, your breathing, and getting the most out of every rep. It must take precedence over lifting heavier and heavier weight and assuming that you are advancing. For example, if a compound exercise for the chest, such as an incline barbell bench press, isn't growing your chest, try doing an isolation exercise such as a cable flye to spark new and noticeable growth.

One thing you'll notice is the most muscular guys in the gym may not be doing much weight but instead are doing their weight of choice very effectively and in a controlled fashion. They're thinking into the muscles and not just moving heavy weight for the sake of moving it.

Changing your routine too often

Not seeing results quickly is the number one reason I see others constantly changing their routines. They may think that the workout they've done only three or four times should be giving them noticeable results. If it doesn't, they feel they're doing something wrong and need to swap out those exercises for new ones. This cycle continues and the muscles never get a chance to truly grow. This can also start to happen if you've been training for years and you're not seeing the same growth and change as when you first started lifting.

It's important to understand that muscles will take more and more progressive overload to continue to grow. Someone new to lifting will see much quicker results with the same effort you apply to your workouts. Simply put, if your routine is working, don't change it.

Maximize each rep

Along with the way you apply mental focus, the way an exercise is performed is also important. During each and every exercise, you must find the balance between time under tension and maximum tension. This means finding the area between your one-rep max and a weight that allows for too many reps.

For hypertrophy to build muscle size, this is typically around 70 percent of your one-rep max. To safely find your one rep max, find the heaviest weight that you can lift four to six times and use this equation (1RM X 1.1307) + 0.6998. For instance, if you can shoulder press 80 pounds for four to six reps, plug 80 into the 1RM section of the equation. This would mean that your one rep max is around 90 pounds. I suggest using this equation instead of attempting to find your one rep max by experimenting with too much weight and injuring yourself in the process.

Training for Results

One major mistake I made for years was doing workouts solely for a pump and not for progression of my overall body. A pump workout is spent essentially doing a randomized and unplanned workout consisting of exercises that pump up your muscles. An example of this is doing a variety of curls and push-ups in one workout until the muscles are pumped. This pumped feeling comes from an increase of blood in the muscle as well as the lactic acid produced as a byproduct of the exercises. This can be okay if you are traveling and just need to do something in a gym that doesn't have your usual equipment. Otherwise, your workouts should be preplanned and part of a progression of weights and reps.

Workout gloves

You may have seen people using lifting gloves and have decided that you need to wear them. In my opinion, wearing gloves will keep your hands from forming the calluses they need for exercises such as pull-ups and deadlifts. There's also nothing like feeling your hands in direct contact with the bar or dumbbell. Some say the gloves provide more grip and are sanitary, but most workout gloves are fingerless so you are still in direct contact with the equipment. Wearing gloves can cause what you are holding to slip, and you are also adding an extra layer between you and the object. I don't recommend them for beginners.

First set syndrome

This happens when your muscles struggle during the first set, giving you a wrong impression of how your future sets will go in that workout. First set syndrome typically happens to me on my first working set of bench press where I am only able to do four reps compared to the 10 that I did previously and the muscles feel weak. During the second set, I am back to where I need to be and the rest of the workout goes fine. Sometimes your first rep can seem shaky and unstable, too, while the second rep is normal and controlled.

Warming up

I'll never start a workout without at least five minutes of warming up the targeted muscle and surrounding muscles. If I start the back workout with lat pulldowns, I'll start very light for 25 reps, then heavier for 15, and then another set just a bit heavier for 10–12 reps. My first working set, or set at my intended weight, begins only after I feel like I am thoroughly warmed up. For biceps, a good indicator that I am warm is when I can see the veins in my biceps and forearms start to fill up with blood. Be careful not to go too heavy for too many sets in your warm-up or it will cut into your strength for your working sets.

Lifting light

The feeling of lifting a lighter weight more times versus lifting heavier weight fewer times is a totally different sensation. The amount of exertion is also much different for a heavy lift compared to the endurance needed for a high rep lift. Your form should always stay as perfect as possible doing either type of routine. For high reps, the form can start to slip and you may rush the last few reps just to finish faster. There is no need to rush your reps or see the final rep as a sort of finish line. For lower reps and higher weight, make sure you are able to give 100 percent. If you fall short of finishing your goal, lower the amount of weight lifted.

Negatives

For years, I thought that doing only the negative portion of a lift during some of my workouts gave the muscles more growth potential. I believed that taking advantage of the slow negative would give me better results. I later learned the only way your muscles benefit from the slower negative is if the weight is higher than the weight you lift concentrically or "on the up phase." This is achieved by having a workout partner assist you on the way up with an exercise such as a bench press. Then the partner lets you lower the weight slowly by yourself, stepping in if it lowers too quickly.

You can lower and control a much heavier weight in the negative phase than concentric phase. Some other examples of this are having your partner help you do extra weight on a lat pull-down, long bar curl, and shoulder press. Your partner can also apply more weight to the negative phase while you are lifting your normal weight. On a bench press, your partner can push the bar down to add more resistance or press down on your hands during a dumbbell curl.

On the flip side, you can make the concentric portion of the lift harder by adding bands, which stretch throughout the lift, recruiting more muscle fibers as the band stretches. You can also get rid of the bands immediately after the set and continue the lift to muscle failure.

Pre-exhaust

This technique can be used for letting the large muscle groups do the bulk of the work and keeping smaller muscles from carrying the bulk of the load. An example of this would be fatiguing the rear delts before an exercise such as a pull-up. Or by doing an exercise such as rear cable flyes for a set of 15 before performing the pull-up, the rear shoulders won't assist as much, thus making the back do more of the work. Use pre-exhaust for the chest by doing triceps pushdowns before your bench pressing or biceps curls before your chin-ups for instance.

Rep timing

Typically, weights are lifted for one second up and two seconds down with max contraction at the top, but you can do all reps slower during one workout or faster for another. You can change this up every workout if you choose; there is no fixed timing for reps. You may decide to do every rep as five seconds up and five seconds down, three seconds up and one second down, or two seconds up and three seconds down. Get creative.

Changing Things Up

As you progress along your journey, you'll want to change some of your lifting sessions through advanced groupings of exercises to shock new growth into the muscles. I recommend trying this after the first eight months to a year of starting your journey.

The first grouping is the giant set, which consists of doing three exercises for a single body part, changing the angle or stimulus on the muscle. Rest time is around 5–10 seconds between exercises with two minutes maximum rest time between the groupings of three. An example of a giant set for chest is an incline dumbbell press, standing cable flyes, and push-ups with your hands on the bench and feet on the floor. Shoot for reps of 8–10. Set up each station before starting the workout, but make sure you are not holding up equipment from other people in the gym.

The second grouping involves pyramid sets. A pyramid is a series of raising reps and lowering the amount of weight lifted over three or four sets and then returning back to where you started. An example would be performing eight curls with 15-pound dumbbells and then 10 curls with 12-pound dumbbells. Next, you would do one more set of curls with 10-pound dumbbells for 15 reps. To finish, proceed down, doing the set of 10 and then the set of eight.

Rest

The amount of rest you'll need between sets depends on the exercise being performed. Typically, lower rep exercises require much more time for recovery. These types of exercises are also typically higher in intensity. Higher rep sets, on the other hand, are normally less intense. Simply put, the harder the exercise, the more rest required.

Usually exercises for legs require the most rest but, for example, squats will require more rest time than leg extensions. For arms, bench press needs more rest than lateral raises. Any bit of rest is helpful, but you want to be fully recovered between sets. For strength training sets of 8–10 reps, rest times of between 45–60 seconds should suffice. Resting for more than two minutes can seem like an eternity. You don't want to get "cold" so try to keep the body warm and moving. Time spent setting up the next exercise usually counts as rest time. If someone is talking to you and making your rest periods go longer than you'd prefer, politely tell them you have to get back to your workout and put your headphones back in.

Rest between workouts

The general consensus for resting between workouts of the same body part is 48 hours, but I think it depends on the level of intensity and body parts trained during the previous workout. Keeping similar muscles from being worked back to back during the week prevents the tired muscles from affecting your next workout. Giving your joints, ligaments, and tendons a rest also have long-term benefits by keeping you injury free.

Workout length

Though there's no set workout time, I suggest you keep your workouts to under an hour. The length of a workout depends on the number of exercises, how long it takes to complete those exercises, and the rest time in between. Bathroom breaks, quick chats with others in the gym, and the length of your warm-up all factor into total workout time. If you are working diligently and not engaging in two-minute conversations after every set, an hour should be plenty of time, no matter what body part you're training. That said, don't worry about workout time, focus on doing what you need to do and not wasting time.

Changing your routine

You never want to reach a plateau and deciding when—and also how—to change your routine is important. While I can't tell you exactly when to change up your routine, there are some basic guidelines. I generally suggest changing your routine at the most every four to six weeks or whenever you stop seeing results.

Some changes include upping the intensity of each set, switching exercises for the same body part, and changing which days you work certain muscles. I also suggest combining compound and isolation exercises of the same muscle right after each other in the same workout. You can also employ using only negatives, drop sets, doing all reps slow, and changing the order of your exercises to mix things up.

Changing up your routine sparks new growth in your muscles. You don't want to switch up the routine any more frequently than four to six weeks because you'll never be able to record when the muscles are growing stronger and your weight is going up. If your workout doesn't leave you with that rush, the feeling like you really accomplished something, and your body got a good workout, it may be time to switch things up.

Training with the proper intensity is very important for many reasons. As you go along, your body will be able to handle more and more intensity. When it comes to lifting weights, intensity can be applied many ways, depending on the exercise you are doing or the body part you are working.

As I mentioned earlier, you'll experience more intensity with legs than any other lift. When going up in weight on squats, for example, the intensity required to push through becomes more and more necessary. Increasing your intensity can also skew your form. You never want to have bad form just to push yourself that extra bit harder. Some will say it's okay to have bad form on the last rep, but those last reps add up over time and can cause you injuries. There's a fine line of pushing yourself to that next level of intensity but also not hurting yourself.

For the chest, for example, you could do 25 push-ups after every set to boost the intensity of the workout, but you could also push out extra reps that totally max you out on every set. You'll also find your energy level differs from day to day, so one day's intense will be nothing compared to the next session when you find you'll be able to go as hard as you can. Remember, though, this should not happen in your initial training stages.

Paying Attention

You may notice that you naturally hold your breath during strenuous exercises. This is the body's natural reaction to getting through the intense portion of an exercise, but you must train yourself how to breathe properly for each lift. The heavier you go with an exercise, the more of importance this becomes. Regardless of the exercise, you must learn to breathe out during the exertion portion and inhale in between.

The phrase "out with exertion" always helps me remember to do this. For an exercise such as dumbbell curls or lat pulldowns, this breathing will seem odd at first. The natural inclination for a curl, for example, is to inhale as the dumbbell comes towards you, but it's important to resist that urge.

Proper form

I wish I had known enough about form to have prevented an injury whose effects lasted for almost 10 years. When performing exercises such as a squat, lunge, deadlift, etc., you must always keep your back straight and protected. This is done by staying in a neutral position with a flat back aligned with your head and neck.

Engaging your core can also assist in protecting the back. I cringe when I see other guys at the gym bending and arching their back to get up out of a squat or deadlift, and they're lucky that they don't blow out the discs in their back.

CHAPTER 13

STAYING THE COURSE

Breaking through plateaus

At some point, you are bound to reach a plateau where you aren't getting stronger or your muscles aren't making the same gains they originally did. The first six months to a year of beginning your strength training can show remarkable benefits, but the law of diminishing returns comes into play and slows that down. Simply put, it takes more to get more.

You can expect to gain about half a pound of muscle a week if you are eating and lifting right that first year. You'll gain more results in the first six months of starting your journey, dropping to roughly a quarter pound per week the second year. When the routine you are following stops giving you results, it's time to change it. This can be done by changing the amount of sets, reps, and tempo of each exercise.

If you have consistently been doing sets of 10 reps, try going up in weight and dropping reps to 8 or lowering the weight and doing 12–15 reps. It also might be a good idea to reanalyze your form for each exercise to see if a few tweaks can help you feel more in the targeted muscle. In terms of tempo, doing reps extra slowly, or pausing at the bottom or top of each movement, can make a big difference in how much you feel the exercise and how many more muscle fibers are kicking in to help finish the lift. Another way to break past a plateau is to find new ways of motivating yourself.

Motivation

Staying on the path of getting stronger and building muscle requires daily motivation and continuing to stay motivated throughout your journey. Sometimes before every workout, I'll stop and reexamine what it is that motivates and drives me to push myself harder and harder.

I also think about why I started my personal journey while I'm warming up. My journey has been a struggle at almost every step, but each morning I wake up wanting to get to the ideal body I have always desired. Some questions I ask myself are, "What or who am I doing this for? Why is it important to do this workout? Will it move me ahead, and what look am I really striving to achieve?"

Your reasons to get in shape will change over time, but a deep emotional drive will keep you going back for more results. Nothing is more motivating than looking in the mirror and seeing the fruits of your hard work, which comes with making smart choices and doing the right things day after day. On those days when you really don't feel like working out, just going to the gym can be enough to make you feel motivated. Having a workout partner is also a huge motivator because you won't let the other person skip the workout, and you're both there to push one other when you're working out.

The truth is, sometimes when you feel like stopping, it just means it's time to start.

CHAPTER 14

TRAIL MIX WON'T CUT IT

When it comes to maximizing your results, nutrition is key. Working out more often and lifting more weight will change your body's makeup, but without following a nutrition program, you will never have the results you are genetically capable of achieving. Following the basic nutrition principles and ideas laid out in this chapter will accelerate your muscle growth, make you feel better, and keep your body changing for the better in the years ahead. (As a side note, I do recommend seeing a registered dietitian in your area who can track what you are eating and give you a plan of specifically what to eat.)

Staying consistent with nutrition doesn't have to be a complicated chore. Eating great tasting snacks and meals will keep you from losing discipline and stopping for that hamburger, fries, and soft drink at the local fast food joint. In this chapter, we'll discuss everything from what to eat, when to eat it, eating on a budget, food preparation, and ways to make overall nutrition as simple and easy as possible. Refer to this chapter frequently to make sure you are accurately following beneficial nutrition guidelines.

Macronutrients

Before we get into what and when to eat, it's important to first understand three basic areas: Carbohydrates, protein, and fat. You must also know how their amounts in each meal and snack applies to what you are eating. Carbohydrates, protein, and fat can all be described as "macronutrients" or "macros." Together, macros are the three ways the body gets energy, and they can only be attained by eating foods that contain them.

Protein

Protein makes up the building blocks of your muscles and provides your body with the amino acids it needs to prevent muscle breakdown. At the same time, protein aids muscle recovery and growth. Simply put, protein is for rebuilding and repairing. For most men, the minimum recommended daily intake is about 56 grams per day, but weightlifters need more, even up to 1 gram per pound of bodyweight. The amount of protein needed to keep the body running daily is about 0.8 grams for every kilogram of bodyweight, which equates to about 1.2–2 grams per kilogram or 0.36 grams per pound. (You can determine your weight in kilograms by dividing your weight in pounds by 2.2). Weightlifters, on the other hand, need about 2 grams per kilo of their bodyweight in protein. One gram of protein is equivalent to 4 calories, and protein should comprise 10–35 percent of your daily caloric intake.

The body can only process between 25–30 grams of protein per hour. If you eat most of your daily protein during one meal, you miss out on its effects throughout your day. Aim for 20–30 grams at every meal and incorporate protein into your snacks as well. Eating the proper protein before a workout is vitally important. Great sources for pre-workout protein are whey, yellow pea, and rice powder shakes with the latter as a great alternative for those with dairy allergies. Foods high in protein include eggs, beef, chicken, cottage cheese, and lentils.

Carbohydrates

Carbohydrates are your body's main food source because they're broken down into glucose and are used as fuel. They can be classified in two ways: Simple and complex carbs. Simply known as sugars, simple carbs are not all unhealthy. Simple carbs are digested and absorbed more easily and quickly than complex carbs. They also contain very little to no vitamins, minerals, or fiber. Unlike complex carbs, they're typically refined and stripped of their nutrients. White bread, French fries, and white rice are all examples of refined simple carbs.

For a quick rule of thumb, if a carb comes directly from nature, it's inherently healthy; if it's processed (changed by man-made processes), it isn't good for you. Examples of good simple carbs are vegetables, apples, oranges, bananas, strawberries, and milk. Bad simple carbs include soda, sweets, cakes, cookies, and candy. The recommended daily allowance or RDA for carbs is 135 grams, which equates to about 45–65 percent of daily total calories. Unlike fat, 1 gram of carbs is equal to 4 calories.

Complex carbs, on the other hand, pack a nutrient punch and include a higher fiber content than simple carbs, which makes them more filling. Complex carbs in the natural state or unrefined state are usually healthy. Some examples of complex healthy unrefined carbs are whole wheat pasta, brown rice, quinoa, potatoes, and vegetables.

For quick reference, good carbs are:
- High in nutrients
- Low in sodium
- Low in calories
- High in fiber

Examples: water, almond milk, low fat Greek yogurt, sweet potatoes, whole grain cereals, quinoa (a starchy seed)

Bad carbs are:

- Low in nutrients
- High in sodium
- High in calories
- Low in fiber
  Examples: juice, soda, lemonade, white bread, white pasta, sweetened cereals, chips, candy bars, syrup, brown sugar, honey

Fat

Fat is a critical source of fuel for the body and a form of energy storage in the body. Your body turns to fat for energy when adequate carbs are not available. Your diet should be comprised of 20–35 percent fat, which equates to about 40–70 grams per day. One gram of fat is equal to 9 calories. Fat also plays a vital role in absorbing vitamins A, D, E, and K into the bloodstream. There are four types of fats: saturated, polyunsaturated, mono-saturated, and trans-fats.

It's important to consume only minimal quantities of saturated fat. You'll find it in milk, cheese, and meat as well as butter, cakes, cookies, sour cream, and ice cream. Saturated fat has been known to increase blood cholesterol levels and the risk for heart disease when consumed in excess. To meet your goals, you want to stay as healthy as possible and avoid caving into treats that contain saturated fat.

Consider:

- Mono-saturated and polyunsaturated fats are easily identifiable because they're in liquid form at room temperature. They're also the "healthy" fats and can help lower LDL or "bad" cholesterol. Examples of mono-saturated fats include almonds, cashews, olive oil, canola oil, avocado, and almond butters.

- Polyunsaturated fats include tofu, walnuts, seeds, salmon, trout, and sardines.
- Trans-fats or trans-fatty acids should be avoided completely. They're fats that have been changed by hydrogenation to make them last longer, and they're found in processed foods and snack foods such as pie crust, potato chips, and microwave popcorn.

For quick reference:

If you are building muscle, shoot for 45–60 percent of your daily diet from carbs, 25–35 percent from protein, and 15–25 percent from fat.

If you are trying to lose weight, shoot for 10-30 percent from carbs, 40–50 percent from protein and 30–40 percent from fat.

Pre-workout Nutrition

Simply put, nutrition can make or break your workouts. If you want as much energy as possible and to get the most out of what you just did in the gym, you must consume the correct foods. Before every workout, you need to know what to eat and when to eat it. If you don't eat the proper foods before your workout, you could get low blood sugar and become dizzy or lightheaded. If that happens, you won't be able to train at the proper intensity or duration required to make the body grow.

Pre-workout snack

Arming yourself with the knowledge of what to eat and when to eat before your workout is critical for furthering your workout success. Your snack of choice should be high in carbohydrates, moderate in protein, and low in fat.

For a rough estimate, you can use your hand to determine the amounts of macronutrients for a pre-workout snack. Carbohydrates, or "carbs," should fill your palm, protein half a palm, and fat, a quarter palm. Since fat is slow digesting, you want to limit it in your pre-workout snack. Instead of feeling energetic, you will likely feel more sluggish. If you're training legs or doing higher intensity for a certain muscle group, it's okay to increase your carbs and boost calories for the workout.

If you are trying to lose weight, shoot for 150 calories with your snack. If you're trying to gain weight, aim for up to 300–400 calories. Often, you won't be heading directly from home to the gym. Because of this, you'll need to have snacks available so you are not working out on an empty stomach. You can keep something as simple as a pack of mixed nuts in your glove box, a pack of rice cakes and a small jar of peanut butter in your desk, or a protein bar in your gym bag as a backup.

Pre-workout snack timing

For snacks, anywhere from 15–45 minutes before the workout is the optimal window to eat. Everyone is different, so finding the right snack and time will take some experimentation to figure out what works best for you. If you're trying to put on weight and mass, it may be a good idea to have a snack on top of having already eaten a pre-workout meal. It's important to time your workouts to occur before or after breakfast, lunch, or dinner.

Here are some other examples of pre-workout snacks:

- ½ cup oatmeal with half or whole sliced banana, almonds, and/or walnuts
- 1 sliced apple with 1 tablespoon of nut butter
- 1-2 rice cakes with 1 tablespoon of nut butter
- 15 baby carrots and 2 tablespoons of hummus
- ¾ cup of Greek yogurt with ½ cup of berries and one tablespoon granola
- Sliced hard-boiled egg with avocado on wheat toast

If you are planning to eat roughly an hour before training, a smoothie can be a great option because it can be digested more quickly than solid food. You can find many pre-workout smoothie recipes available online.

Here's one example:

(You may have to experiment with blending times/ amount of milk to reach your preferred consistency.)

- ½ cup milk or almond milk
- 1 scoop protein powder
- Handful of spinach
- 1 cup frozen berries
- 1 scoop of flax seeds or chia seeds

Pre-workout meal

Consuming a snack before a workout is perfectly fine but ideally, you should eat a meal. Also, a pre-workout meal can be even more important than the post one. The meal should be around half the portion size of your typical breakfast, lunch, and dinner. It's meant to give you a boost of energy. The optimal time to consume this meal is one to two hours before training since you don't want anything remaining in the digestive tract; you want it available to your muscles.

Your pre-workout meal should be easily digestible but it doesn't have to be fully digested to begin giving you energy benefits. Having a substantial pre-workout meal can prevent muscle breakdown and encourage muscle growth.

The meal should be roughly 400–500 calories and contain a good source of protein, healthy fats, and carbs. Shoot for around 20 grams or approximately 4–8 ounces of fast digesting protein and a complex carb (beans, vegetables, whole grains) of around 20–30 grams or roughly 1 ounce.

As far as healthy fats go, such as avocado or olive oil drizzled over the meal, shoot for 1 tablespoon. Since fat is slow to digest, use it in lower amounts for this meal and higher amounts in your other meals.

To better or more accurately determine protein for your meal, multiply your weight in kilograms by 0.2 grams. To find your weight in kilograms, divide your weight by 2.2. For a 150-pound man, his weight in kilograms is roughly 68 and his protein requirement is about 13 grams. For carbs, divide your weight in pounds by 2.2 and then multiply that number by 0.5.

Here are some examples of pre-workout meals:

- 4 oz. salmon with 4 oz. sweet potato, green beans, and 1 tablespoon olive oil
- 4 oz. chicken breast, brown rice, and broccoli with accompanying healthy fat such as olive oil.
- 1 can of tuna mixed in a bowl with ½ cup hand crushed whole grain crackers and mustard, pepper, and relish to taste
- Oatmeal with a scoop of whey or pea protein mixed in and 1 banana
- 4 oz. of chicken with sweet potato, asparagus, and olive oil
- Cooked egg whites on a plain bagel

Pre-workout meal timing

The optimal time for a pre-workout meal is one to three hours before your workout. Ideally, try to eat within three hours of the workout. As with a snack, you may have to experiment with different meals and times to determine what is best for you. Eating the meal sufficiently before or after your workout allows for better digestion and nutrients to be adequately absorbed. A large meal sitting in your stomach too close to the workout can cause digestive issues. If it has been more than three hours since you ate a meal, you should eat a snack.

Post-workout Nutrition

Just as critical as a pre-workout meal or snack is what you eat when the workout is over. The body has an increased need for nutrients post-workout, and growth is dependent on what you feed it. You must always eat post-exercise, even if all you have available is a small portion of nuts or a pack of crackers. Anything is better than nothing. Along with your pre-workout snack or meal, you should be prepared and know what you are going to eat afterwards. In particular, you want carbs that can be digested quickly, which is important for enhancing recovery.

Post- workout snack

Try to eat snacks within 20–30 minutes if you are unable to eat a meal, since this is your optimal window to gain benefits. You should still have protein from the pre-workout snack or meal working in your body. You can eat within two hours and still receive benefits, but after a workout, the sooner you eat, the better. Also, a convenient snack or meal will make you more likely to eat. An easy option is a shaker bottle with milk and protein powder chilled in a cooler or lunch box during your workout.

You want your post-workout snack to contain carbs that can be digested quickly. Since you'll be doing strength workouts, make sure you have enough protein in your pre-workout snack. Egg whites, chicken, turkey, low fat cheeses, Greek yogurt, and nuts, such as cashews and almonds, are all good ideas.

Here are some ideas for post-workout snacks:
- 2 hardboiled eggs with a slice of whole grain toast
- 1 slice of whole grain toast with 1 tablespoon of nut butter and ½ a banana
- 1 cup of chocolate milk
- Greek yogurt and mixed berries
- Orange slices and almonds

- Trail mix (dried banana, nuts, raisins, dried cranberries, sunflower seeds)
- Shake of 12–16 oz. of milk/almond milk with 1 scoop of protein powder

Post-workout meal

A post-workout meal should pack a punch nutrient-wise, just like a post-workout snack. You can time this meal to coincide with your breakfast, lunch, or dinner. As with snacks, timing is critical. Options for post-workout meal proteins are tofu, beans, fish, turkey, and chicken. Ideally, carbs should be quinoa, brown rice, nuts, or whole wheat bread. For macros, a combo of about 30–60 grams of carbohydrates, up to 20 grams of protein, and just a bit of fat (5–8 grams).

Here are some examples of post-workout meals:

- 4 oz. of steamed trout with a baked sweet potato and sautéed spinach
- 4 oz. grilled chicken and 1 cup mixed vegetables
- 1 cup oatmeal, banana, whey protein, and sliced almonds
- Wheat toast with 2 scrambled eggs
- Whole grain wrap with 4 oz. chicken
- Bowl with 1 chicken breast, 1 cup brown rice, 1 cup veggies

Drinking Water

Along with diet, it's imperative to stay properly hydrated inside and outside the gym. Drinking enough water before a workout is important to prevent cramps and dehydration. You should also drink water throughout your workout, about one cup every half hour.

During your workout, it helps to have a shaker bottle full of water or your water bottle nearby to limit leaving equipment and/

or waiting in line at the water fountain. Even mild dehydration can impact your workout. Drinking water also helps flush toxic byproducts out of your system. Make sure you drink throughout the day and not just a large amount at once. For daily hydration, aim for half your body weight in ounces of water.

It's an excellent goal to shoot for one gallon of water a day. A clean gallon milk jug with a screw-on cap is a cheap option, or you can purchase a large water container to help ensure you get the full amount for the day. If you use a milk jug, you can mark times on the side to make sure you're drinking it evenly throughout the day. For example, writing 9:00 a.m., 12:00 p.m., and 4:00 p.m. keeps you from over or under drinking. You can also add a slight flavor to your water, such as lemon.

You can gauge whether you are hydrated enough by the color of your urine, especially when you first wake up. It should be almost clear unless you are taking a multivitamin. Water-soluble vitamins in a multivitamin are flushed from your body and can cause coloration.

Meals

Now that you know what to eat before and after workouts, what should you eat for your other meals? It depends on whether you want to lose or gain weight. The number of calories you consume can make or break your muscle growth. To gain size, you must eat! It's imperative that you take in the necessary number of calories. This means eating often and eating the right type of foods.

To put on weight, you need additional calories because your body burns them as part of its natural energy processes. This is called your Basal Metabolic Rate (BMR). On top of this, you have your Total Daily Energy Expenditure, which combines BMR with your energy expenditure throughout the day. If you are highly active, you'll need the excess calories to help put on weight. If you're on your feet moving around all day, your body is burning even more calories. Ideally, you want to shoot for 1–2 pounds of weight gain per week.

To calculate your BMR, use the formula below:

- (To find weight in kg, divide weight in pounds by 2.2.)
- (1 inch = 2.54 centimeters)

BMR = 66 + (13.7 x weight in kg) + (5 x height in cm) – (6.8 x age in years)

To calculate your Total Daily Energy Expenditure, (TDEE), use the following equations. This is the number of calories you will need to maintain weight. You'll need to eat at least 400–500 calories on top of this number to gain weight and at least 400–500 less calories to lose weight.

Sedentary	
Little or no exercise, job requires long hours sitting	TDEE = 1.2 x BMR
Lightly active	
Light exercise	TDEE = 1.375 x BMR
Moderately active	
Moderately active	TDEE = 1.55 x BMR
Very active	
Heavy exercise	TDEE = 1.725 x BMR
Extremely active	
Very heavy exercise, physical job, training 2 times per day	TDEE = 1.9 x BMR

When you're trying to build muscle size, multiply your weight by 15 to calculate the calories you need. For instance, a 130-pound male would need approximately 1,950 calories. Based on this chart, you also need a calorie surplus in order to grow, but don't go too far because it will turn to fat. More eating means more volume and more frequent training.

If you're not gaining weight, bump up your daily calories by 100 or cut back on the amount of cardio.

There are three different body types—ectomorph (thin, fast metabolism), mesomorph (athletic build, easy gainer), endomorph (overweight, very slow metabolism)—and they determine your caloric needs. If you are trying to lose weight, modify each snack and meal to slightly smaller portions. If you're trying to gain weight, you can add extra portion sizes or follow these guidelines. If you're trying to maintain weight but put on muscle, follow these guidelines closely or slightly reduce the portions.

Breakfast

For starters, you want to eat in the morning at least 15–30 minutes after waking. Breakfast is a vital meal, especially if you plan to work out in the morning.

Ectomorph Choose any option:

Meal 1
- 1 cup oatmeal, 1 tablespoon nut butter
- 1 banana or 10 strawberries
- 3 scrambled eggs
- (Optional) glass of whole milk or almond milk

Meal 2 (breakfast smoothie, great for on-the-go)
- 1 cup yogurt or whole milk
- 1 cup oats
- 1 tablespoon nut butter
- 1 cup frozen fruit or berries

Meal 3
- 1 cup cottage cheese
- 1 cup fruit and berries
- 2 pieces of toast with 2 tablespoons nut butter

Meal 4
- 1 cup oatmeal
- 1 scoop whey powder

- 1 banana or apple
- 1 glass whole milk

Meal 5

- 3 eggs
- 2 pieces of toast
- 1 banana
- 1 glass of whole milk

Lunch

Meal 1

- 6 oz. chicken
- 4.5 oz. brown rice
- ½ cup black beans
- 1 cup vegetables

Meal 2

- 5 oz. of ground beef
- 1 large potato
- Shredded salad

Dinner (Choose any option for meal)

Meal 1

- 5 oz. steak
- 1 cup yellow potatoes
- 1 cup cooked asparagus
- Glass whole milk

Meal 2

- 5 oz. chicken
- 1 cup cooked asparagus
- 1 tablespoon olive oil

Meal 3

- 1 cup mixed greens
- ½ cup chickpeas

- 2 tablespoons dressing
- 5 oz. chicken
- 1 medium sweet potato

Meal 4

- 5 oz. salmon
- 4.5 oz. brown rice
- 1 cup cooked broccoli

Meal 5

- 5 oz. tofu
- 4.5 oz. brown rice
- 1 cup cooked asparagus

Meal 6

- 5 oz. 93 percent lean beef
- 1 large sweet potato
- 1 cup mixed veggies, cooked

Eating on a budget

Buying the amount of food you need on a weekly basis can be expensive, but there are ways to get the calories you need without breaking the bank. For starters, look to buy the majority of your food at a warehouse club that offers more bang for your buck. You can purchase large quantities of brown rice, peanut butter, eggs, oils, and produce while saving money at the same time. Get the bulk of your calories from these foods as well.

Try not to go out to eat; you can make the same meals at home a lot more cheaply. It's also helpful, no matter where you shop, to purchase generic brands over brand name foods. Generic brands are usually very close in taste and texture to brand name foods. Take advantage of store sales and use coupons, if possible. Lastly, buy large bags of food like frozen veggies, which are just as nutritious, tasty, and fresh.

Food Prep

Cooking your food ahead of time is important for consistency of progress towards your goal. You must stay as consistent with your eating as you are with your training. Knowing what you are going to eat for the day/week keeps you on track and should be preplanned, just like your workouts. The next section will walk you through the food prep process and keep you from becoming overwhelmed with the thought of making all of your meals at one time.

Start slowly. If you just want to prep only lunches for the week, that is fine. Be sure that all of your meals are simple but tasty. If you have a recipe you really like, keep it in a special binder where you can easily locate it to make it again. Eating food throughout the week that you don't enjoy will only push you closer to cheating on your nutritional requirements.

Planning

You have to choose meals and the day(s) you are going to prepare or prep your food. Typically, Sunday is the best day to prep because you'll be ready for the week. Prepare to spend about two hours getting everything ready. If you know you have a work lunch/dinner or will need to skip a meal for any other reason, factor this into the amount of meals you are making. I suggest blocking out prep time in your schedule each week to make sure you are able to get everything made.

You can prepare meals for the entire week on Sunday, but food will start to have an altered taste about four days later, and it may be bland or soggy. If you don't enjoy what you're eating, you're more likely to grab something else, such as fast food or a sugary snack from the convenience store. The foods you choose should be tasty and enjoyable and not just be consumed as fuel. It may take a few weeks to determine what tastes best when reheated and what stays fresh three or four days after preparation.

Shopping

The first step of food prep is buying your food for the week. Make a grocery list by writing down each meal and its ingredients. Stick to this list when shopping, and don't shop when you're hungry because you'll be more inclined to make impulse buys. Before heading to the store, check your list against what you already have at home.

You can also order your groceries online, if possible, and pick them up at the store or have them delivered.

When shopping, I'd suggest not buying fresh veggies, fresh fruit, or meat in bulk because of how quickly they spoil. For fresh veggies, I suggest buying them precut to save time during prep. You can also purchase frozen veggies in large quantities, which are flash frozen upon picking and contain the same nutrients as fresh veggies but last a lot longer. For more flavor to your meals, I also suggest purchasing salt-free spices.

Prepping

Once you have everything needed for your daily meals, it's time to chop it, steam it, cook it, and organize it. Multitasking makes the process go much faster. While something is cooking in the oven, you can have a pot on the stove, something in the microwave, and a cutting board to chop veggies all going at once. Start the longer cooking items first and do the rest of your prep while they're cooking.

When the cooking is completed, you can either put each item into its own container or you can put a full meal into each one. If you already have containers, make sure you have all the lids. If your containers and lids are too mismatched, I suggest buying new containers to lessen confusion and frustration. Opt for glass over plastic, which can warp in the dishwasher and is more environmentally friendly. If you use plastic containers, make sure they're BPA free. I also suggest picking up some masking tape to label each container.

For quicker cooking options, opt for microwave rice pouches and cups that can be tossed together with canned tuna or chicken for a tasty pre- and post-workout meal. Also, cooking a large batch of quinoa provides an easy add-on option for meals or salads.

Purchase bags that allow you to carry your meals anywhere and have a place for your shaker bottles. These are especially convenient because they come with containers and are lined with insulation to keep meals cold during transport.

Some of you may prefer crockpot cooking to standard stovetop and oven cooking. With crockpot recipes, your food is ready for you at the end of the day, and you can use leftovers for the next day's lunch and dinner.

Cheat Meals

The phrase "cheat meal" gets thrown around a lot in the fitness community, implying a meal that gives you a break from your daily routine and is typically something such as pizza or chicken wings. It's best to refer to this meal as a "treat" meal instead, as the word "cheat" makes it seem like something you should not be doing.

A treat meal can be most helpful as a psychological break from your eating routine and can also help boost your metabolism. The problem with these meals is it is easy to overdo it and one piece of pizza can turn it into five pieces, leaving you feeling bloated and sluggish the next day. A treat meal can also turn into a treat day, taking your calorie intake way above what it should be. My suggestion is to have a small portion of your intended treat meal in addition to your normal food for the day.

You'll want to continue to refer back to this chapter to adjust what you are eating and make sure you're getting the best results possible. Starting out your journey with a solid nutritional foundation will provide benefits for years to come.

CHAPTER 15

SUPPLEMENTS

As a beginner, you may wonder what supplements are and how they can affect your results. Keep in mind, growth will occur without supplements but taking them can move you along to your desired physique much faster. The ones I cover in the following sections include protein powder, creatine, BCAAs, and pre-workout powders. There are many other types of supplements, but I think these are the most important ones.

Protein powder

It's always best to get your proteins from food but extra protein can help boost your results, especially after a workout. Most people are familiar with whey protein powder. There are other types of protein powders, and finding the right one for you will take some time. If you're lactose intolerant, or need a gluten-free option, you'll find you have many choices. At most supplement stores, such as Vitamin Shoppe and GNC, you'll typically find soy, hemp, pea, and other vegan protein powders.

Mass gainer supplements tend to be front and center when you walk into most supplement stores. These are typically very high in calories and contain a large amount of carbs and protein and are usually recommended for the ectomorph body type. If you are not a hard gainer, these are all right but will pack more fat on you than muscle. For most protein powders, the more you pay, the higher quality item you'll get. I'd suggest reading reviews before you make a purchase.

If you're on the go or don't have a meal planned right after a workout session, a protein shake is the way to go. Many people mix their protein with water in a shaker bottle, but I don't recommend this. If you happen to find one that mixes well with water and has a decent taste, go for it, but most taste better and mix best with almond, coconut, or regular milk.

Be sure you have a quality shaker bottle with a mixer ball or some other way to break up the clumps. There's nothing worse than getting a big clump of dry protein powder. Also, be sure not to leave a shaker bottle in a hot car because when you open it up to rinse it out, you may not care to smell it. I also suggest the shaker bottle option because if you blend your shake in a blender, it may become too foamy and undrinkable. For extra calories and health benefits, you can add things to your protein shake such as flax seed oil, chia seeds, and MCT oil.

Creatine

This is another popular supplement that has gained notoriety in the fitness world over the past 30 years. Overall, creatine in the form of creatine monohydrate is the number one supplement choice for athletes and lifters. It's known to increase strength as well as improve muscle mass. To understand how creatine works, let's take a more scientific look.

Muscles get energy for lifting weights through a molecule called ATP, or adenosine triphosphate. This is a chain of three phosphates attached to adenine. When the third phosphate on the chain of three releases, energy is released, powering a muscle contraction. Throughout your workout set, ATP in the muscle diminishes. After the first rep of your set, the stored energy covers the rep, but since your body only uses the third phosphate, the two remaining phosphates are left, which is called adenosine diphosphate. The two remaining phosphates combine with creatine phosphate, turning on ATP again and powering the intended muscles.

If the supply of creatine phosphate is depleted, your body jumps to the anaerobic system, which doesn't supply the same amount of power as creatine. This extra supply of creatine phosphate comes from keeping the creatine storage tanks full by supplementing with creatine monohydrate. Creatine monohydrate comes in pill as well as powder form. Some suggest mixing it with a high glucose drink to help it reach the cell more quickly but drinking water will work just fine. I recommend taking 5 grams per day with a large glass of water.

Some foods like beef and chicken contain creatine, but consumption of these foods alone doesn't give you enough grams. Although your body can naturally synthesize creatine, taking extra creatine has been shown to increase power output but won't solely increase muscle mass. More muscle mass will be attained with being able to lift more weight through your sets by having extra energy during your sets. Creatine also makes your body retain water, which can look like more muscle.

BCAAs

I suggest BCAAs, or branch chain amino acids, for everyone from beginner to advanced lifters for the extra energy boost they can provide during a workout and also for their ability to help slow the breakdown of muscle. They have also been shown to help with delayed onset muscle soreness, which can be intense soreness two days after a workout.

Branch chain amino acids are essential amino acids, which means your body can't make them itself and they must be consumed. What are amino acids? They're simply the building blocks of protein with each one serving a specific function. There are three amino acids that make up BCAAs: Isoleucine, which helps with energy uptake, preserves protein breakdown, and helps your body use fatty acids; valine, which the body can use for fuel when glycogen stores are low; and leucine, which helps preserve lean mass, increases insulin levels, and activates mTOR, which promotes muscle growth through protein synthesis.

These three amino acids can be found in daily foods. Good sources of leucine in foods are eggs, soy, and fish. Isoleucine is found in eggs, many seeds, and fish. Valine is commonly found in eggs and soy as well as elk. You may not need to purchase BCAAs as a standalone supplement because many protein powders already contain them. Also, 30 grams of protein from beef or a scoop of protein powder contains around 6 grams of BCAA. In general, eating enough dietary protein is sufficient for your daily BCAA intake.

BCAAs typically come in a powder or pill form and can be taken before, during, and/or after the workout. I suggest adding to your water bottle.

Pre-workout supplements

Pre-workout is a generic term for powder supplements that include caffeine, beta-alanine, l-citrulline, and BCAAs combined into one. These ingredients provide a boost of energy and work as vasodilators. A vasodilator opens your blood vessels to allow more blood flow and gives you the "pump" during your workout. Caffeine is the main stimulant in most pre-workouts, many of which have the equivalent of three or more cups of coffee. Some also come without caffeine.

One of my favorite benefits of pre-workout is that it can give you the extra motivation you need to start your workout. Sometimes if you are not feeling like working out, the pre-workout can get you fired up when its effects kick in. I usually take it about 30 minutes before my workout with 8–12 ounces of water, or whatever is recommended on the label. If the label says that you may take one to two scoops, start with a half a scoop and see how it makes you feel during the workout.

Certain workouts, such as legs, can make you shake or become nauseous if you do them while on pre-workout due to the already elevated heart rate. Don't take pre-workout if you are going to be doing cardio at the gym, as it will only raise your already elevated heart rate.

CHAPTER 16

YOUR FIRST WORKOUT

It's time to get to the gym. First, prepare your food then decide when you are going to do your workout. If you plan to work out early in the morning, you might be a bit excited and ready to. You may also wake up and just want to go back to sleep. Finding the best time to go to the gym will take some trial and error, and every day will be different. You may be motivated or able to train at 8:00 a.m. some days, but on other days you won't be ready until lunch time, a work break, or after dinner.

How do you know what part of the body to work when you get to the gym? I've set out chapters on each body part, a full list of exercises, and easy-to-follow workouts. You'll also find a guide about weight and how to increase it safely. Be sure to read each chapter in detail so you are fully prepared to get right to work when you enter the gym.

Also, it's important to be familiar with the equipment you're planning to use. Having a plan in place before walking into the gym makes your workout go more smoothly and you can get in and out without wasting any time. You'll want to track all of your workouts, especially the first one, using a workout log that can be purchased online ahead of time.

Walk into the gym with confidence and get right to work. Make sure you have a filled water bottle from home. That way you don't have to worry about warm water from a water fountain or waiting in line between sets. Time wasted at the gym will hurt your results. Within weeks you will be seen by others as the guy who knows exactly what he is doing and you'll fit right in.

One good idea is to write or print out your workout beforehand so you know exactly what you will be doing. It might change, however; for instance, you could be ready to do flat bench press or flat dumbbell press and no bench is available. You may need to do a longer warm-up while you wait if this is your first exercise. You can sub in another exercise and do that instead. Plan to keep your workout under one hour, and if done with all of your sets, plan plenty of time to stretch afterward.

Which warm-up should you do before the workout? It depends on your body part. If it's cold outside, be sure to properly warm up so you don't have cold muscles, especially if you're rushed into your workout. If you are working out with a workout buddy, make sure they know to be on time. Also, make sure they have their own workout log so they aren't writing their numbers in yours.

If you choose to use a gym bag, make sure you don't bring it onto the gym floor. As discussed earlier, many gyms have rules against this because it can get in the way of other gym-goers and is also a trip hazard. You can keep your gym bag in a locker, but first check to see if your gym has them. Some have paid options and locks to borrow; others are free if you use your own lock.

In your gym bag, be sure to have your workout clothes if you plan to change into them after work. You don't want to be psyched up for a workout only to get to the gym and not have a change of clothes. Once you've picked out a few different shirts and a couple pairs of good shorts and pants, you won't have to purchase much else. Be sure to keep a clean pair of clothes in your car as backup in case what you have on isn't fresh or if you have forgotten your gym clothes. Wash your gym clothes inside out to clean them well. And be sure not to wear cologne since some people may have allergies and you may be working out in tight quarters.

Also make sure you have the right pair of shoes. You never want to enter a gym for your workout wearing dress shoes or flip-flops.

Here are some packing tips:

Gym bag. Bringing a gym bag with you to work out is a great idea so you have one place to keep everything you need. If you plan to shower at the gym, make sure to pack flip-flops for foot health. Also, pack a pair of clean clothes and socks if you plan to shower after your workout. You don't want to change into mostly clean clothes and have to wear one dirty item. I also suggest bringing travel-sized bottles in Ziploc bags for showering.

Bring your headphones and keep a charging cable in the bag in case you need to charge them on the way to the gym. Keep a pair of regular cable headphones in your bag in case your wireless ones go dead or you forget them at home. It's not a bad idea to bring a plastic grocery bag for dirty clothes to contain odor. You can bring a small gym towel with you, ideally one that has a clip or carabiner, so you can hang it from the machine instead of putting it on the floor. You can also bring a lock if you feel uncomfortable leaving your gym bag in an unlocked locker.

Tops. Shirts that fit well for workouts accentuate your upper body and motivate you to become more muscular. Wearing a shirt that is too baggy will make you appear smaller and feel less motivated. What kind should you buy? You'll find a large selection of workout shirts and clothing at your local sporting goods store. I suggest you try to wear sweat-wicking clothes made of polyester and Lycra blends, especially for days when you do leg workouts.

You want to make sure you have room to move in your shirt as well as your workout pants or shorts. Freedom of movement for exercises prevents you from falling and also allows you to go to end range.

Bottoms. For leg workouts, you ideally want to have workout shorts. If it's cold outside, you can put pants over them and then change when you get to the gym. Be careful if your shorts are too long—they can catch around your knees. For workout pants, make sure they can stretch so you have a full range of movement. If you are doing a leg workout, shorts will keep you more comfortable and cooler.

Shoes. A basic pair of athletic shoes is fine but make sure they don't have too much cushioning. The cushion will compress as you do heavier squats and deadlifts, leaving you feeling unsteady.

CHAPTER 17

WORKOUT MACHINES AND EQUIPMENT

Though you shouldn't rely solely on machines for your workouts, you'll need to use them for almost every part of the body at some point. You may wonder, "What's the difference between using machines compared to using free weights?" The answer is simple: machines typically follow a fixed path of motion, unless you are using something that is attached to a cable, such as a bar for lat pulldowns.

Free weights, on the other hand, rely on stabilizers and core strength, in addition to the targeted muscle, to perform the lift or exercise. Muscles are not meant to follow an exact path and being locked into following one can cause strain or injury. Many new gym-goers will flock to exercise machines because they see using them as a quicker workout. They'll usually stick to using these same machines and not see much in the way of results.

Machines have their place in weightlifting, but for your purposes now, you should mostly be using free weights such as barbells and dumbbells. As your workouts change, you'll use them more frequently. Many machines at the gym will be unfamiliar at first, but most have simple instructions printed on the side. Some machines may have directions for a few exercises, but this is no substitute for knowing how to set up the machine and understanding the proper form for doing the exercise.

If it's an upper body machine, make sure it doesn't feel awkward or that a certain angle causes shoulder pain or discomfort. If you still are unsure how to use it, watch someone else using the machine. Gauge their height and overall size, along with the machine settings and the weight they use. For lower body machines, the placement of your body as well as the setup of the machine will determine the effectiveness of the exercise and whether you could end up hurting yourself. Machines are not meant to be used quickly because this can cause injury as well.

COMMON GYM MACHINES

Smith machine

The Smith machine is a guided barbell that moves up and down. You can apply weight on either end for exercises, such as bench press or squats. The barbell moves along a track, and a frame on the outside of the bar has hooks that allow the bar to lock into place before or after your set. The Smith machine is used by many beginners to start bench pressing and squatting because it guides the arms or lower body and provides safety catches in case you are unable to finish the repetition.

The main reason this machine is criticized is that the stabilizer muscles don't assist as they would in a regular bench press and squat. One advantage of the Smith is that it's good to use without a spotter because the weight can be racked at any point, compared to a bench press or squat bar that can only be racked at the top of the movement. The Smith machine may allow you to lift heavier weight than you can with free weights, but don't be fooled by trying the same weight and hurting yourself using free weights.

For advanced weightlifters, the Smith can be a great way to finish out muscles to full fatigue using high reps or going to failure without worrying about the weight causing injury. Intermediate and advanced lifters prefer it for exercises such as seated and standing calf raises as well as shrugs because of the smaller movement path. The Smith machine can be used facing forward or backward for exercises such as squats and lunges, but you'll want to see which way you prefer racking and un-racking the bar. Racking the bar by twisting the wrists forward versus backward can be extra tricky during specific exercises.

Cable crossover machine

The cable crossover machine can be found in most gyms and usually comes with other attachment areas, such as a lat pulldown or a place for seated rows. Each side of the machine has cables that can move up or down a vertical rail. They raise and lower by pulling back a plunger handle and releasing it to lock-in when you've set it to the predetermined weight number. Each hole has a number so you can make sure each side is at the same level. Attached to the cables are carabiners or clips that allow for the attachment of D-rings or accessories such as V-handles or a small straight bar.

Even though this is a machine, the motion is entirely free. It uses your stabilizer muscles because the cable attachments are on a pulley piece that freely swings side to side. Exercises such as cable flyes are a great way to build the chest and can only be achieved using this setup. The ability to use all different heights of the cable columns allows you to change the angle of this exercise, working the muscle in many different ways.

One issue you might run into with this machine is that someone will already be using one side, forcing you to choose another exercise if you need both sides. When using a cable machine of any type, make sure it moves smoothly on both sides. You don't want one side to be struggling to move while the other side is fluid and free.

Also, check to make sure the cable is correctly attached to the weight plates and that your attachment is securely clipped. Sometimes the carabiner or clip won't be straight. It can become stuck, and you'll be able to pull the weight, but during the lift, the clip can slip into its proper position causing a jolt that may cause injury.

Leg press

The leg press is a heavy-duty staple at most gyms, and usually there is more than one. To use, you lay on it, putting your feet up at an angle on a wide foot plate and push the weight along a fixed path. This is a great alternative for men who have problems squatting.

I don't recommend using it when you are starting out, or at least not for your heavy leg exercise. You can use the leg press for finishing the legs out with high reps. The standard leg press can be loaded with weight plates, or there is another version that allows you to sit upright and put a pin in the stack of weights so that you can choose the weight.

One problem with leg press machines is that people will put their feet too low and their knees end up going way over the toes as they lower the machine to the bottom. The leg press should mimic a squat, and the knees should stay in line with the toes. Another problem with the leg press is that some people will lift their lower back off the back pad and twist to get the weight up if it's too heavy. Don't do this. It can cause back issues as well as leg injuries.

Also, be sure when using a leg press to set the safety catch in case you can't lift the weight back up so it won't come down and injure you. A big no-no with the leg press is to leave it stacked with the plates you used. You'll often come upon a leg press that has eight or more 45-pound plates on each side and you have to remove them all just to start your workout. (See Chapter 11 for more details about gym etiquette.)

Lat pulldown machine

The lat pulldown machine is an essential part of any gym. Many lifters like to use it in place of pull-ups if they're able to do more than 10 pull-ups easily and need weight to help the latissimus muscle continue to grow. The machine typically has a cushioned seat and circular roller pads that help lock you in place, helping you feel secure to achieve more reps.

Various handles can be attached to the lat pulldown machine, but you'll mostly be using the long bar attachment, which mimics a pull-up. Other machines create a lat pulldown effect using levered bars that allow weight plates to be added; these are called convergent machines. They follow a fixed path compared to the lat pulldown, which allows forward or backward body movement when you set up for the exercise or when a slight form change is needed for the last couple of reps.

Leg extension/leg curl

The leg extension and leg curl are two widely debated machines. Some lifters don't use them because they don't allow the body to move as it naturally should. During a leg extension you are seated and only your quad muscles move the weighted pad up and down. This is unnatural because your glutes and core are not engaged to help move the weight. The same is true for the hamstring machine, whether it's the seated version or the version that has you laying down. Because only the hamstrings and calves are used to some degree, your body is locked into an unnatural motion.

Machine Safety

Some machines may appear to be in working order but actually are not safe. How do you tell? First of all, you'll see that adjustment levers don't lock into place well. If something isn't locked in, it can pop loose, causing a quick jerk and possibly tearing a muscle. This quick force can also snap a cable, causing weight plates to drop and possibly hurt you or someone else near the machine. If you attempt to lock a setting of a machine into place and it's rusted out or doesn't click into place, skip the machine altogether.

Expanding Your Horizons

You can learn about many more machines than are listed here. When the gym isn't busy, take your time learning to use them and configuring the setup that works best for you. Some machines, such as a leg extension, can have multiple adjustments with each one affecting the other. Machines such as a pec deck flye machine and seated chest press can be complicated to adjust. Don't try to set them up for the first time when the gym is busy while others are waiting for it.

Machines have their place and as you progress, you'll find yourself using more of them and discover new ways of using them beyond simply basic use. Turning a different direction and then pulling or pushing the machine handles can change the exercise or even the targeted body part. You'll find yourself experimenting once you have used the machine multiple times or seen someone else using it differently. Try to mimic what they did or ask them for a quick review.

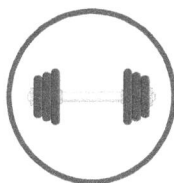

PART 4:
FOCUSED TREKS

CHAPTER 18

HOW TO TRAIN YOUR CHEST

The chest, along with the arms, are the two most visible and highly trained body parts, and they get the most attention from others.

"How much do you bench?" is a question that applies to the flat bench press exercise, the standard for chest strength. The flat bench press works mostly the middle of the chest and can neglect upper and lower chest muscles. Many guys start their chest workouts with flat bench press and add an incline bench press as their second or third exercise.

Your chest workout should begin with an incline bench press or incline dumbbell press. Bench presses use a barbell, and the advantage of using dumbbells is to build up the chest evenly. Sometimes one arm can do more of the work, which makes it stronger and more dominant. Dumbbells, on the other hand, allow each limb to work independently along with improving your independent limb control. They also allow for a broader range of motion.

Dumbbells can become harder to hold as you go up in weight, and you don't want your grip to hold you back from getting stronger. Grip strength is vital in many other exercises, but you want to make sure it allows you to focus on chest building. You don't want to worry whether or not you will drop a dumbbell on yourself as your grip weakens throughout the set. (See Chapter 18 for an in-depth guide to building your grip strength.) When using a barbell, minimal grip strength is required, though it's beneficial to have a firm grip in weightlifting overall.

Another fundamental exercise for working the chest is the push-up. Doing more than 10 push-ups in a set won't build much muscle, but you can add resistance in the form of a weight vest or use push-ups at the end of your workout to burn out the chest. Using all sorts of different angles for hand placement during push-ups or placing one hand on a ball or an unstable object during the push-up can shock new growth into the chest.

By performing an alternate type of push-up, your repetitions may drop so they can be used for muscle growth sets. Using push-up handles, stationary or rotating, can be an excellent exercise for the chest and more beneficial than flat push-ups on the ground. The ability to go below the handles stresses the chest more to build more muscle. Flat push-ups tend to put too much pressure on the wrist and their range of motion is limited by the chest touching the floor. If push-ups on the ground hurt your wrist or you don't own push-up handles, you can use a dumbbell set on the floor holding the handles in place of a push-up handle. That way, you'll keep the wrists in a much more stable and comfortable position.

There are many different exercises that you will use to train the chest and different variations of how those exercises will be completed. I suggest thoroughly looking up each one of the following exercises and how to do them on the American College of Exercise's video library to see them appropriately performed. The website can be found at https://www.acefitness.org/education-and-resources/lifestyle/exercise-library/video.

The goal in chest training is to not only grow muscle and create a great looking physique overall but to also get stronger. For bench press, the milestones for strength are being able to bench press 135 pounds, 225 pounds, and 315 pounds. It can take a considerable amount of time to reach each of these numbers. Along with a muscular chest, you must also have strong shoulders, triceps, and grip strength as well as a strong core to be able to complete the lift. There's nothing like the first time you can lift one 45-pound plate on each side (135 pounds) or two plates for 225 pounds and three for 315 pounds

Exercises for the chest include:
- Flat Dumbbell Chest Press
- Incline Dumbbell Chest Press
- Decline Dumbbell Chest Press
- Flat Bench Press
- Incline Bench Press
- Decline Bench Press
- Flat Push-ups
- Incline Push-ups
- Decline Push-ups
- Bar Dips
- Cable Flyes

You'll want to start easy with chest training and work your way up to more weight and adding exercises. Your endurance will increase with each workout. As your strength goes up, your body will adjust to the routine. At first, the workouts laid out in this chapter may seem too easy. Keep your chest workouts to twice a week with three days in between to allow for adequate growth. When the chest is no longer getting sore from a routine, it's time to add sets or an additional exercise. Keep accurate records of your workouts, even if you are only able to perform a total of 10 push-ups for your first workout. Looking back at your numbers and seeing your progress will be a huge source of motivation.

You can do many things to improve your chest workout, which leads to better results. Here are some exercise-specific tips:

Bench pressing

For starters, keep your glutes, hamstrings, and core tightened to make sure you have the most amount of power available for each lift. Having your entire body tight and engaged will give you much more strength. Each time you do a set on the bench press, bring your hands out just a bit wider than you did during the previous set to engage extra muscles in the chest. Also, try not to rest the bar on the chest during each rep, which takes the tension off the chest muscles. Instead stop the bar about an inch above the chest. One way to think about benching is that you are pushing yourself away from the bar and not the bar away from you.

Bench press plateaus

You may encounter a plateau when benching, and one way of breaking past it is using what is called a "dead bench." This is accomplished with a power rack and setting the stop bars slightly above your chest. That way, you push a bench press rep from the bottom and not starting at the top and coming down, causing the bar to stop dead slightly above your chest after each repetition. Building strength at this part of the lift will help you out of the "hole," which is when you are stuck at the bottom and can't move the weight to complete the repetition.

Benching without a spotter

When doing this, you want to make sure the barbell doesn't have clips on each end. Don't worry about the plates sliding off since the weight of the plate combined with the roughness of the bar will keep them from easily sliding. The importance of taking the clips off is to ensure that if you can't get the bar up off you at the bottom of the movement, you can lean the bar to one side or the other and wait for the plates to slide off. Be very careful not to drop plates on someone standing next to you using another machine or hit them with the bar. Once the plates fall off one side, the bar will quickly flip back the other direction, so be ready for this.

Proper elbow position

A key factor to remember when doing any type of bench press, as well as push-ups and dips, is not to let the elbows flare out from your side parallel to your shoulders. Instead pull them in slightly toward your side, saving your shoulders from injury.

Push-ups

When doing push-ups, don't lock out your arms because this will transfer the weight to the joints and off the muscles at the top of the push-up. Use a wider hand placement of your push-up handles for more overall chest activation, moving hands closer together for more triceps and inner chest focus.

Working the chest from every angle

Starting from the top down, the upper chest is worked during an incline bench press at a bench angle of 30–45 percent. The upper chest can be worked at this angle using dumbbells as well as a barbell. To work the middle chest, use a flat bench or one that has a slight incline. To work the lower chest, use a decline bench, preferably one that has pads to lock in your knees and feet. Without these, you may fall off during the lift or strain your low back.

A comparison: bench press, dumbbell press, cable press

Unlike the cable and dumbbell press, the contraction of the chest is limited during barbell presses because the hands can't come together at the top of the press. The benefit of cables is that the hands can be crossed at the end of the movement, further maximizing the chest use compared with dumbbells. The grip use is minimal in a cable chest press, and there is also no risk of dropping a bar or dumbbells on you. The only word of caution I have for you is to slowly lower the handles when you are done so you don't slam the plates together in the machine.

If you're doing dumbbell presses, you must know how to lay back with the dumbbells, especially as they get heavier and heavier. The way you pick up the dumbbells to begin the lift is a matter of personal preference. You may pick them up off the floor while seated on the bench or lift them off the rack each time. Once you have them in your hands, place them vertically on each thigh. Next, kick one knee up towards you, followed by the other leg, as you lay back. This allows the weight of the dumbbells to help you fall into place, ready for the lift to begin. You'll find that dumbbells are harder to handle compared to the same weight on a free bar. The bar is still difficult to hold but it requires less forearm strength to control than a dumbbell in each hand.

Flyes

I prefer the cable flye over the dumbbell flye because there is constant tension on the chest throughout the movement. Cable flyes can be done in a decline, incline, or flat position. I also prefer to use metal D-ring handles versus black vinyl strap handles because the handle rolls with the flye movement. When doing cable flyes, squeeze the pinkies in each hand and try to angle the D-rings at the end part of the flye so that the base of each handle touches to engage the most amount of chest muscle. Also, keep a slightly bent elbow on each arm during cable chest flyes throughout the entire movement.

Pressing properly

Regardless of whether you're doing cable, dumbbell, or barbell presses, think about pressing from the elbows. Keep the hands directly above the elbows at the bottom part of the movement to keep a good stretch on the chest and then drive them forward.

Dips

When performing parallel bar dips, keep the head and back aligned with your spine and lean forward slightly. You may have a tendency to look up and forward during a dip but this is incorrect form. Some parallel bar stations have handles that rotate inward and outward. The outward handle setting is for the chest while the inner bars target the triceps. Keep the elbows extra close by your sides for triceps dips and slightly wide for chest dips.

Before the Workout

Make sure to properly warm up for at least five minutes before starting these workouts, and warm up with each exercise before performing your first set. If you start with incline barbell bench press, for example, start with reps of just the bar weight. If the bar is too heavy to warm up for higher reps, you can do the same exercise with dumbbells.

Use a weight that doesn't fatigue you and starts to give you a slight burn at around 15–20 reps. I recommend performing 2–3 warm-up sets before you begin your starting weight. With each subsequent warm-up set, add 5–10 pounds more on the bar. If this is too much, go up by 2.5 pounds on each side. If your first chest workout is only push-ups, your warm-up can be modified by doing push-ups on your knees or on a higher surface like a workout bench or a Smith machine bar. You can lower or raise the bar on the Smith machine in four- to five-inch increments to change the angle, reducing the exertion needed for a full push-up.

Using dumbbells can help balance you out as well as increase your barbell strength. Before starting one of these workouts, you'll need to identify which weights to use. Start with 7.5 pound dumbbells if you've never done these exercises. If that feels too light, increase the weight to 10 pounds. Make sure to keep your dumbbell weight increases small—for example, from 10s to 12.5s, 12.5s to 15s.

When using a barbell, go up in weight by 5-pound plates each time until the total weight equals a 25-pound or 45-pound plate, for instance. If you're working out at home and need extra weight for push-ups, you can fill a backpack with books and strap it to your back to create a weight vest.

Chest Workouts

Note: You can change these workouts every four to five weeks by altering the order of the first three exercises.

Beginner (1x/week)
Push-ups (on floor/Smith Machine): 3 sets of 8–10 reps, rest 90 seconds
Incline dumbbell press: 2 sets of 8–10 reps, rest 90 seconds
Decline dumbbell press: 2 sets of 8–10 reps, rest 60 seconds
To make the workout more difficult, increase the weight used and lessen the rest time.

Beginner-Intermediate (1x/week)
Incline dumbbell/barbell: 3 sets of 8–10 reps, rest 60 seconds
Decline dumbbell/barbell: 3 sets of 8–10 reps, rest 60 seconds
Flat dumbbell/barbell: 3 sets of 8–10 reps, rest 60 seconds
Push-up: as many as you can do
To make the workout more difficult, increase to 4 sets of each exercise and/or increase the weight.

Beginner-Advanced (1x/week, increase weight for more difficulty)
Incline dumbbell/barbell: 3 sets of 8 reps, rest 45 seconds
Flat dumbbell/barbell: 3 sets of 8 reps, rest 45 seconds
Decline dumbbell/barbell: 3 sets of 8 reps, rest 45 seconds
Incline push-up (hands on a bench, feet on floor): to failure (see Chapter 3 for details)

Intermediate (1x/week)
Incline barbell/dumbbell press: 3 sets of 8 reps, rest 45 seconds
Decline dumbbell/barbell press: 3 sets of 8 reps, rest 45 seconds
Flat dumbbell/barbell press: 3 sets of 8 reps, rest 45 seconds
Flat cable flye: 3 sets of 10 reps, rest 45 seconds
Push-up: to failure (add another set to failure for more difficulty)

Intermediate-Advanced (2x/week)
Incline barbell/dumbbell press: 3sets of 8 reps, rest 45 seconds
Flat barbell/dumbbell press: 3 sets of 8 reps, rest 45 seconds
Dips on parallel bars: 3 sets of 8 reps, 1 minute rest
Cable flyes High to Low: 3 sets of 8 reps, rest 45 seconds
Cable flyes Low to High: 3 sets of 8 reps, rest 45 seconds
Push-up: 25 (any variation; for more difficulty, add weight in the form of a weight belt or weight vest for dips)

Advanced (2x/week)
Incline barbell/dumbbell press: 4 sets of 8 reps, rest 45 seconds
Close grip dumbbell press: on flat bench 3 sets of 8 reps, rest 45 seconds
Parallel bar dip: 3 sets of 8 reps, rest 45 seconds
Feet elevated push-up with 3-second pause at the bottom: 3 sets of 10 reps, rest 30 seconds
Flat cable flyes, seated on bench in middle of cable crossover machine or use flye machine: 3 sets of 10 reps, rest 30 seconds
Incline dumbbell drop set: starting with weight that allows for 15 reps, go to failure, and then drop the weight by 5 pounds and repeat to failure, and then drop one more time.

Helpful Tips

Here are a few things to look out for to avoid sabotaging your chest workout and reducing the chest muscles:

1. Don't let your triceps move too close to the body during any form of bench or dumbbell press, as this will engage the triceps and take the emphasis off the chest. Though the triceps are used to assist in pressing motions, they should not be taking anything from the chest. They should only support it. One way to engage the chest over the triceps is to try to pull the hands towards each other while doing any barbell bench press. This engages the chest a considerable amount and will increase the burn during the lift.

2. Be sure not to train the triceps before your chest day. They'll be weaker because they're sore. As a result, they won't be able to adequately help the chest. The same applies to the shoulders.

3. As you advance, you'll perform the cable flye exercise. Flyes can turn into a press if you have the handles turned the wrong direction. For a proper cable flye, the palms should face each other with a tight grip on the D-ring or handle attachment. When performing the move, lean forward slightly and open the chest so you don't engage the shoulders. Many guys do a rounded bear hug while doing flyes and end up leaving the chest out of the move. Always push the chest out as much as possible during flyes and roll the shoulders back.

4. An inclined, declined, or flat bench press machine usually has the angle set for the lift. If you use a regular bench for dumbbell pressing, make sure it isn't angled up too high. Otherwise, you'll be working more shoulders than chest.

5. One of the biggest mistakes you can make during chest training, or any body part, is to let your mind wander

or lose focus on contraction. As you develop more muscle overall, you'll feel more of a contraction during each movement.

Spotters

A spotter is crucial for keeping you safe. A spotter can also help motivate you in case you can't complete your final few reps in exercises ranging from chest presses and squats to military presses and seated dumbbell presses. A good spotter knows just how much weight to take off, allowing you to complete your rep safely.

At some point, you may be asked or may ask another person in the gym to spot you for one set. Typically, this is when you are trying a one-rep max or hitting a final heavy set of your chosen exercise. You don't want to ask someone to spot for you on two or three consecutive sets, which would take them away from their own workout. Not only will they get annoyed but they will also care less about adequately spotting you.

There are a few different ways to spot someone performing a bench press. To begin, you have to know and understand how to remove just the right amount of weight for them. When spotting a bench press, stand behind the bench with hands placed on the bar slightly inside the lifter's hands. I always prefer to use a switch grip, which means one hand is facing up and the other facing down. Stand slightly behind the end of the bench, being sure not to stand directly over the lifter's face. Lean over slightly while assisting the rep, keeping your core tight to protect your low back.

A proper spotter is only there to help out if needed during the rep. If someone asks you to spot them, they may know they can get the weight up but want you there in case they can't push out the last few inches. Not having to worry gives them greater confidence going into their set. They will need help un-racking the bar from the rack, and you can assist them as much as you want but sometimes they will ask you not to help them.

When they're lowering the bar, keep yourself ready by keeping your hands on the bar in the proper spotting technique described earlier but don't lift or push in any direction. This allows them to control the bar freely. If they drop it, you are right there, ready to assist, and don't have to spring into action if you have your hands off during the descent portion of the lift. If they're unable to get the weight off their chest, be ready to get into position, doing whatever you need to help them lift the weight to the lowest racking position. If you are unable to get the weight off their chest with their assistance, call out to others in the gym to help you.

If you are starting out and are not very strong or well versed in spotting, tell the person you are not comfortable spotting them if they have a lot of weight on the bar. There will be plenty of other people in the gym who are more comfortable spotting that weight, and there's no need for you to get hurt.

If someone begins slowly lifting the weight from their chest and it starts going slower and slower, you know they need your help. Begin raising the bar straight up, not pulling back towards you. If the bar still isn't moving, pull upwards to give them more assistance until they can reach the lowest rack position.

The spotting technique for the military press is similar to bench press, but you are typically standing tall with both hands in the palms-up position. Sometimes military press racks will have foot platforms to raise you higher than the lifter so you can bend over slightly to assist the lift easier.

The spotting technique for dumbbells is different from barbells. Because there is nowhere to grab, like the middle of a barbell, you have to use a different technique. The method I prefer is to press up from their elbows from a slight squat with a flat back or on your knees. The key here is to press up on their elbows and only give as much assistance as needed.

If their weights are too heavy even for you to assist, tell them to dump it. You have a better sense of how much further they have to go in the lift and are almost in control of the situation. If you need them to dump the weights, say it sternly and so they can hear you. Ideally, you can guide the dumbbells back to their chest and allow them to roll up to starting positions and set the weights down. If they need to drop them, make sure others are aware the dumbbells are going to fall and get out of the way. A dumbbell can bounce or roll, especially when dropped fast, and it can crush toes or hit someone during their lift and cause them to drop their weights or injure them.

Going Forward

As you progress with your chest training, you'll want to add new exercises and try more variations to shock growth in the chest. Incorporating machines to isolate a specific part of the chest can help, leading to new muscle growth. You may find yourself wanting to use different machines such as the pec deck and butterfly machine along with new variations using cables. Adding weight through the use of a weight vest or weight belt during dips can also help decrease your reps and build strength at the same time.

Another way to add to your chest workout is to superset another muscle, typically the back. While the chest is resting, the back muscles can perform an exercise. Supersetting allows for more muscle growth for both body parts. Since you'll be doing work when you would usually be resting, you'll want to lengthen your rest time after performing the second exercise of the superset.

The chest can also be a superset with biceps or legs. Supersetting with triceps or shoulders isn't a good idea because you don't want those muscles to wear down when you need them. Some people like to superset chest with abs, but you need all the core strength you can get to perform chest exercises. You don't want your core weakening during the workout. If you choose to do abs, wait until after your chest workout is finished. Also, make sure that a weakened core won't impact your next day's workout.

When you're using a gym while traveling and it has lighter weights than you're accustomed to using, you can create a workout based on doing three to four sets for each part of the chest using the lighter dumbbells and do higher reps. Other ways to use lighter weight include pressing with only one arm at a time without a weight in the other hand or performing reps extra slowly. If nothing else, performing high reps of push-ups in your hotel room can also be a great workout. Try for max reps in one minute, and then attempt to beat your number for four sets in a row.

Regardless of your chest workout, push yourself as hard as possible. Always make sure you're pushing harder than you did the previous workout. You'll feel more comfortable coming up with new workouts as you make progress, and you'll discover there are an infinite number of ways to change things up.

Here are some examples:

- Perform 10 push-ups after every set of any chest exercise.
- Perform as many push-ups as possible in a minute, rest one minute, then repeat 10 times.
- Do a pyramid set. Start with 15 reps and choose a weight, drop down to 12 reps and choose a heavier weight, 10 reps and a heavier weight, and then repeat the set of 12 and set of 15 subsequently.
- Perform a normal rep and then the bottom half of the rep, followed by another normal rep and half rep.
- Perform one exercise with a barbell and then the same exercise using dumbbells.
- Perform pressing dumbbell exercises holding a dumbbell in one hand only (lighter weight) and controlling each rep slowly.
- Perform an upper, lower, and flat chest exercise back-to-back in circuit fashion.

As you go continue, your chest workouts will change in terms of exercises and their reps and sets. You may try a high rep routine if you are starting to do a shred for summer or get in shape for a wedding. Other times, you'll experiment with heavy weight and low reps for strength. There is no "one way" to train the chest. As long as you are pushing yourself and challenging the muscles, you'll experience growth and positive change.

It can be helpful to return to lighter weight to feel the chest fully engaged if you have been going heavier and heavier for growth. You may be building bigger shoulders and not improving your chest size. It's also a good idea to take a picture of your chest each month to see what areas you need to bring up.

Reassess your current routine after a few weeks and see if it's giving you the results you want. Have you gradually switched into doing more isolation exercises when your focus should still be on heavy compound exercises? Have you changed to doing more bodyweight training and your reps have gone too high? If you are training by yourself, is it time to seek out a workout partner to help spot you and push you to get that little extra and break past strength plateaus? These are all questions worth asking to make sure you are on the right track to meet your goals.

CHAPTER 19

HOW TO TRAIN YOUR BACK

The back muscles, like the legs, are typically undertrained. Nor can the back be seen during most back exercises, which can limit the mind-muscle connection required for proper training. Many lifters waste years incorrectly training their back muscles and instead end up growing their arms. They tend to focus on isolation exercises or doing too many reps. A well-developed back is difficult to achieve but is very noticeable with or without clothing.

The main goal with back training is twofold: The first is to create a V-shape taper of your muscles by doing pulldown exercises and making the lats grow wider. For back thickness, the goal is to build by doing rowing motions. Wide lats and a strong, pronounced upper back are not only aesthetically pleasing but functional.

You'll start to notice your shirts fitting tighter because of your growing lats. You'll hear the lats described as "wings," and watching them grow will give you great confidence going into each subsequent workout. For me, pull-ups were what gave me the most results in this department. It also helped to use variations of wide and close grip pull-ups.

The back is used for everything from carrying groceries to lifting your suitcase. You'll definitely notice strength gains as you perform daily tasks that just seem easier. A strong back will also help lift your chest muscles and combat poor posture. Doing pulling movements also helps balance out the pushing movements of chest, shoulder, and triceps exercises.

Like any muscle group, the back requires focusing on every repetition. If you are just going through the motions of the exercise and using momentum to move the weight, you'll never achieve the growth and strength for which you strive. It helps to pause and squeeze every rep at the bottom or top of the motion, depending on the exercise. Also, be careful not to move up in weight too quickly. Master the basics of form and then begin to add new exercises later.

Grip Training

You may see other lifters using straps for back exercises such as deadlifts, rows, lat pulldowns, and pull-ups. These straps take the burden off your grip by wrapping tightly around the bar or object you're holding, keeping it in your hands. Many exercises can't be performed with good form if you don't have grip strength, so lifters bypass that by using straps.

Though many lifters are opposed to them, lifting straps have their benefits, and many beginners depend on them. You can use straps starting out but I don't advise it. You'll miss out on the forearm and grip strength development that you'll desperately need as you progressively get stronger.

Grip strength will happen naturally as you do more lifting and increase the weight, but training your grip and forearms on your off days can also help. Purchasing grippers that vary in weight or even rolling up a towel and squeezing it for a period of 30 seconds to a few minutes can build up your endurance so your grip and forearms don't fail you before your back can get a proper pump during training. Metal grippers are measured in pounds and allow for reps, much like regular lifting. The target muscle for these are the forearm flexors. I don't suggest you buy plastic grippers because they become too easy too fast, unless you are beginning with zero grip strength starting out.

You can also work on your grip at any time using a lighter gripper, but treat the heavier grippers as a workout using sets and reps. You can use a lighter gripper while stopped at a stoplight or watching TV, performing reps to failure or until your hand cramps.

For the opposite muscles of the forearms, the extensors, you can use bands that wrap around all five fingers. I had to buy these because of pain I experienced while assisting my workout partner during a bench press. For some reason, as soon as I finished helping lift the weight, I had a painful cramp in the top of my forearms that would last for about 30 seconds after every set. Strengthening my extensors fixed this. These muscles don't get a lot of attention but they are important.

Pull-ups

The pull-up is an essential compound back exercise, especially since it also works the biceps, forearms, shoulders, and core. If you struggle with doing even one pull-up or chin-up, don't worry. I'll explain how to build up so you can perform 10 in a row.

You can work up to performing your first pull-up in various ways. Using a lat pulldown machine and upping the weight weekly can help you gain enough strength to do one pull-up. To do this, sit down and bring the knee pads to your thighs at a level where you feel secure and locked in. Make sure your feet are flat on the floor. Finding the right weight can be tricky during your first workout but start lighter for warm-up sets with higher reps.

Breathe out as you pull down with a big breath in on the way up.

Don't let it slam down after completing your set, as the weights can break. Lean back just slightly; it should mimic a pull-up, and there should be no momentum during the pulling down phase. Also, don't go too wide or use any grip that feels uncomfortable. While the lat pulldown may isolate your lats well, your body will become stronger and more fit overall by doing pull-ups.

To do a pull-up negative, simply place a step below a pull-up bar at a height that allows you to grip the bar without straining your arms. Next, jump up off the step or whatever you are standing on until your chin is above the bar. Make sure not to bend your head back to achieve a higher chin. Place your palms on the bar so that they're facing away from you slightly wider than shoulder width with your thumb on the same side as the other fingers.

If you're performing a chin-up, use the opposite hand position, palms facing you. You can also work up to chin-ups using this same method. They work more of the biceps than a standard pull-up but are a great addition to a back workout. Once you have mastered pull-ups, you may find yourself being able to do 10 chin-ups as well.

Another way to perform both a chin-up and pull-up is to use an assistive banded device. These clip onto the bar and have a foot attachment with multiple bands that take weight off your body. As you get stronger, you can remove a band and eventually work your way to not having to use any.

Some gyms will have something called an assistive pull-up machine. This is a standard pull-up station equipped with multiple grips and two foot holds to help you get up to the bar. Attached to the device is a fold-out platform that is typically padded. At the bottom of the machine is a stack of weight plates that can be adjusted with a pin. The weight in this stack is the total weight taken off your body during the assisted pull-up.

The attachment is used by folding it out so it's parallel to the floor and locked. When you rest your knees on it during the pull-ups or stand on it (if it's able to go low enough), you will be lifted with the assistance of your chosen weight. As you get stronger, you can reduce the weight of the plates until you are able to do pull-ups without them.

It will take time but incorporating pull-ups and chin-ups into your routine will help you achieve your desired physique even faster. They're key to upper body strength and essential to building a solid, powerful, and defined back. As you advance, you can add weight to pull-ups with a weight belt or other method but only if the back is doing all of the work and not forcing the arms to work harder.

Look for overall back muscle growth and strength at the start of your training. Don't be concerned with growing a specific back muscle through advanced training methods and isolation. The top back exercises for building the most size and strength are deadlifts, wide grip lat pulldowns, and rows.

Some lifters like to do similar exercises together. For example, they do pull-ups followed by a lat pulldown variation and then move to one arm rows and bent over barbell rows. You don't have to do this starting out, but you may choose to arrange exercises in that order as you progress.

I recommend watching videos on the ACE Fitness video library website at https://www.acefitness.org/education-and-resources/lifestyle/exercise-library/video or seeing live training demonstrations for each of the following exercises so you can hear a detailed explanation and witness proper form. Reading how to do them in a book or listening to them on an audiobook can also give you some idea of how they're performed, but nothing compares to seeing them with your own eyes.

An exercise like a deadlift has a lot of moving parts, and it must be performed correctly for safety and maximizing muscle growth as well as using the proper muscles to achieve the lift. Not understanding one cue in instructions can lead to injury so be sure you understand the ins-and-outs of any workout you perform.

Exercises to grow a strong and impressive back include:
- Barbell deadlift
- Pull-up
- Chin-up
- Wide grip lat pulldown
- Close grip lat pulldown
- Overhand barbell row
- Underhand barbell row
- Two handle pulldown
- Hyperextension
- Single arm dumbbell row
- Seated cable row
- Dumbbell shrug
- Barbell shrug

Before Working Out

Make sure to warm up but don't exhaust yourself. A good way to warm up the back is by performing reps of light lat pulldowns before pull-ups. Other methods include light reps of rows, some push-ups, and large arm circles. Never rush your warm-up; it's a critical part of any workout. If you're starting with deadlifts, load up about half of your body weight, or intended first set weight, and perform 15–25 slow reps.

You also have to figure out your starting weight for each exercise. If it's your first time, start out very light to be sure you are using proper form. Jot down the exact weight for each exercise in your workout log and track your progress from the start. I made the mistake for years of not writing my weights down and repeated workouts using the same weight as the previous workout—or lighter, in some cases.

The proper starting weight for you will be different from everyone else. Regardless of your weight, make sure that the last one to two reps of your sets can be completed, though not with ease. If you're twisting your hips, neck, or torso to complete the rep, the weight is too heavy. If you find yourself shifting your body around or using bad form on the third of four reps, you are definitely going too heavy.

If you are going up in weight on an exercise such as a lat pulldown, for example, and the next weight plate is just a bit too heavy, you can go back to your original weight. Some gyms will have a 5-pound piece of hardened metal covered in rubber made specifically to rest on top of the top weight plate in a machine stack, adding less weight than the next plate on the machine. Another way to add weight if this piece isn't available is a 2.5- or 5-pound plate resting on the weight pin if the end of the pin is able to hold it. Though this is technically not advised by the machine manufacturers, it's a way to add a bit more weight as long as the pin is still able to go all the way through the weight plates safely.

Other Options

If you're working out at home, I recommend purchasing a multi-grip pull-up bar that fits in your doorway. Make sure it's sturdy and will be able to hold your weight, even with a weighted backpack or weight vest. If you have a solid workout bench, you can use it for single arm dumbbell rows. If you don't own a barbell and only have a set of dumbbells, you can use them in place of barbell exercises, such as underhand rows and shrugs.

My recommended gym workouts can be modified for your home gym. As always, be sure to write down in your weight journal how you modified a certain exercise so you can repeat it during the next workout.

Unilateral Training

Unilateral training, or using one arm at a time, also can be a great and effective way to strengthen a lagging back muscle. During exercises such as pull-ups and barbell rows, both arms are working, and if one is stronger or one side of the back is stronger, that side will continue to stay dominant. Using one arm at a time allows you to restore balance and make sure each arm is able to do the same amount of weight and reps.

Some advanced lifters like to break up their back training into two days separated by two or three days. These sessions typically focus on exercises such as pulldown variations, pull-ups, and straight arm pushdowns to grow their back wider. On thickness days, they focus primarily on rowing motions.

The workouts in this chapter can be modified as you progress and made more difficult by the addition of more sets, reps, and heavier weight. The use of free weights should be fundamental to your back training but adding in machines as you advance will help build even more muscle.

Important safety notes:

- Before doing deadlifts, I suggest you thoroughly warm up the lower body as well as the upper body because of many muscles used during the exercise.
- Don't shorten the range of motion on chin-ups and don't rest at the top either, keep tension throughout the movement.
- Always do lat pulldowns in front of your head towards the top of the chest. Don't lean too far back, as it will turn the pulldown into a row.
- Keep your chin just slightly lifted, but don't lean the head

all the way back to stare up at the bar.

- Retract the shoulder blades back and down each set to get an extra squeeze/contraction.
- Place the thumb on the top side of the bar next to the fingers (thumb-less grip).
- When using the lat pulldown machine, bring the knee pads down as tight as you can on top of your legs to lock you in place.
- Drive your feet into the floor or foot placements so you don't lose tension during the exercise.
- During the seated cable row, sit up tall and keep the core tight. Retract the shoulder blades back before each set and during the set to get an extra squeeze. Place your feet on the rubber foot pads with a slight bend in the knees, bring bar to the chest. Thumb-less grip is advised on these as well.
- For the one arm flat bench dumbbell row, raise and lower the weight at the same tempo, making sure not to jerk the weight up. Keep the chin down, make sure the back of the head is aligned with the back. Perform this parallel to a mirror, if possible, to check your form or have a workout partner check it for you.
- Try to isolate the back on every back exercise, mentally try to let the back, and not the arm, do the lifting.
- For bent over barbell rows, the underhand, or supinated grip, allows more natural motion and more range of motion. Be careful when un-racking the bar for this in a supinated grip, start it on a rack so you don't have to lift the bar off the floor every time.
- A neutral grip, where the palms are facing towards your sides, is going to be your strongest grip.
- Don't straighten arms at end of a row, for risk of tearing

the biceps.

- Straight arm push downs are better performed while kneeling. When doing a straight arm wide pushdown, pretend to pull the hands apart which will engage the lats.

- The back is stronger arched than flat, which is why it may try to arch during certain exercises, but don't let it.

- Make sure to do back exercises in the mirror so you can see yourself from the side, or film yourself and go back to watch and check.

- A deadlift alternative is using a hyperextension machine, angled higher than flat to make it more difficult. To increase hyperextension difficulty, hold a weight plate at the chest.

- Don't let the back round during deadlifts

- Use a trap bar instead of barbell for the deadlifts if available at your gym.

- If you have wrist issues, you can use an EZ bar for your underhand rows.

- If, as your deadlifts get heavier, you find that they zap your strength for later exercises, add them into the workout as a later set. Since they require so much muscle use to perform, they can weaken the lats, traps, and rhomboids as well as grip and forearms.

- You can use straps for shrugs, either dumbbell or barbell. The range of motion is much better with dumbbells but it becomes harder to hold heavy dumbbells compared to the bar.

- Much like the barbell or dumbbell row, make it easy to grab your shrug weights so you aren't bending down every set.

Workouts

Beginner (1x/week)
Lat pulldown: 3 sets of 10 reps, rest 45–60 seconds
Seated cable row with lat pulldown bar (palms down): 3 sets of 10 reps, rest 45–60 seconds
One arm bench dumbbell row (palm facing your side, doing each arm back-to-back before resting): 3 sets of 10 reps, rest 45–60 seconds
Straight arm pushdown using lat pulldown bar: 3 sets of 10 reps, rest 45–60 seconds
Hyperextension: 2 sets of 10 reps, rest 30 seconds

Beginner-Intermediate (1x/week)
Deadlift with barbell or trap bar: 3 sets of 8 reps, rest 45–60 seconds
Lat pulldown: 3 sets of 8 reps, rest 45 seconds
Flat bench dumbbell row: 3 sets of 8 reps, rest 45–60 seconds
Dumbbell shrug: 3 sets of 8 reps, rest 45 seconds
Hyperextension: 3 sets of 10 reps, rest 45 seconds

Beginner-Advanced (1x/week)
Deadlift with barbell or trap bar: 3 sets of 8 reps, rest 60 seconds
Pull-up: 2 sets of 8 reps, rest 60 seconds
Lat pulldown (if unable to do pull-ups): 8 reps of 3 sets, rest 45–60 seconds
Seated cable row (2 handles or V-handle): 3 sets of 8 reps, rest 45–60 seconds
Dumbbell shrug: 3 sets of 8 reps, rest 45 seconds
Hyperextension: 2 sets of 10 reps, rest 30 seconds

Intermediate (1-2x/week)
Deadlift: 4 sets of 8 reps, rest 60 seconds
Pull-up or lat pulldown: 4 sets of 8 reps, rest 60 seconds
One arm flat bench dumbbell row: 3 sets of 8 reps, rest 60 seconds
Inverted row on Smith machine bar: 3 sets of 8 reps, rest 60 seconds
Dumbbell or barbell shrug: 4 sets of 8 reps, rest 45 seconds
Hyperextension: 3 sets of 8 reps, rest 45 seconds

Intermediate-Advanced (2x/week)
Deadlift: 4 sets of 6–8 reps, rest 60 seconds
Pull-up: 4 sets of 8 reps, rest 45 seconds
Inverted row on Smith machine bar: 2 sets of 10
Dumbbell or barbell shrug: 3 sets of 8 reps, rest 45 seconds
Underhand barbell row: 3 sets of 8 reps, rest 45–60 seconds

Advanced (2x/week)
(Deadlifts or pull-ups can be done in any order, so feel free to change them around.)
Deadlift: 4 sets of 6–8 reps, rest 60 seconds
Pull-up: 4 sets of 8–10 reps, rest 45 seconds
Underhand barbell row: 3 sets of 8–10 reps, rest 45 seconds
Seated cable row with two handles: 3 sets of 8–10 reps, rest 45–60 seconds
Dumbbell or barbell shrug: 3 sets of 8 reps, rest 45 seconds
Hyperextension holding 25-pound plate at chest: 3 sets of 15 reps, rest 45 seconds

CHAPTER 20

HOW TO TRAIN YOUR SHOULDERS

Shoulders, or delts, are vanity muscles like the biceps and easy to see in the mirror while you're training. Shoulders look great when well developed and building what is called a "cap" that creates a broad, wide look. Having strong shoulders also will assist you on many other exercises.

Starting out, you'll perform mostly compound lifts for the shoulders. Don't be worried about isolation exercises or about shaping the deltoids. Ways to work the shoulders include barbells, dumbbells, and cables. The key to training shoulders is to maintain tension on the muscles throughout the entire movement, regardless of whether you're working front, middle, or rear delts.

The front delts will grow faster than the others because they are used in exercises including dips, chest presses, and bench presses. The rear delts are also worked during pull-ups to a small degree. Having strong rear deltoids is important to slow down a bench press. A lot of guys undertrain the rear delts because of the small amount of exercise it takes to properly work them.

The following workouts will be your keys to building size and strength. Shoulders can be worked without a spotter since the dumbbells can be dumped, if needed. If your gym has a military press machine, this will help. But doing a seated shoulder press with dumbbells will work fine too.

There are all sorts of variations on shoulder exercises such as doing a shoulder press with a twist at the top, doing them individually, or holding tension on the bottom part of the movement and then performing the press. Bands are also a great way to exercise the shoulders and are helpful on side raises or doing rear delt work.

Exercises for shoulders include:
- Military press
- Seated dumbbell press
- Dumbbell lateral raise
- Rear dumbbell flyes
- Dumbbell side lateral raise
- Upright rows

Important safety notes:
- Make sure the triceps doesn't take over on rear delt work, don't bend the arm a lot to keep this from happening.
- A common mistake I see is during side raises, the arms are locked out or bent too much. There should be a slight bend at the elbow for a standard side lateral raise, and make sure the wrists are not turned up or slack down. Don't bring the hands together at the top of the movement, instead pressing the dumbbells straight up from where they start and returning to that same position.
- When doing a military or dumbbell press, press through your feet, make sure knees are bent but push into the ground to give yourself force through the whole body.
- I have taken out front raises because the front delts are used in so many extra exercises, and you don't want to waste your gym time overworking or overdeveloping a muscle.
- When isolating the middle delt and not letting the traps and front shoulders do the work.

- For seated and standing shoulder presses, bring inside of dumbbell directly above top of shoulder.
- Don't let arms slack at top of shoulder press, the joint is very unstable in this position.
- Better stability on seated shoulder presses than standing, barely bend arms to keep tension, press all the way to rest and then do more reps.
- Wider position on upright rows, the more shoulders it works and less the traps.

Workouts

Beginner

(Note: I suggest doing your shoulder presses and side raises standing when you are a beginner to build core stability with glutes tight as you press the weight. As you move up in weight, you may find yourself arching the back to complete the move. This is especially important on a push press, which is a standing barbell press.)

Standing dumbbell shoulder press: 3 sets of 10

Standing dumbbell side raise: 3 sets of 10

Rear dumbbell flye: 3 sets of 10

Beginner-Intermediate

Seated dumbbell shoulder press: 3 sets of 10

Standing dumbbell side raise: 3 sets of 10

Rear dumbbell flye: 3 sets of 12

Intermediate

Seated military press: 3 sets of 10

Standing cable side raise: 3 sets of 10

Upright barbell row: 2 sets of 10

Rear cable station flye: 3 sets of 10

Intermediate-Advanced
Seated military press: 4 sets of 8–10
Seated dumbbell side raise: 4 sets of 8–10
Barbell upright row: 3 sets 8–10
Bent over rear cable flye: 3 sets of 10–12

Advanced
Seated military press: 4 sets of 8
Seated dumbbell side lateral raise: 4 sets of 8
Rear cable flye: 4 sets of 8
Upright row: 4 sets of 8
Seated dumbbell press: to failure

CHAPTER 21

HOW TO TRAIN YOUR ARMS

Training your arms refers to building your biceps and triceps. To many guys, this is the most rewarding workout because of the pump that's achieved very early in the workout. A biceps curl superset with triceps pushdowns can create a quick visual reward. Being able to see and feel the pump drives you into pushing harder and harder and gives you the sensation of watching your muscles grow right before your eyes. Though their appearance dissipates after the workout, the memory of how they looked in the mirror will keep you coming back for more.

When it comes to training arms, you can try many exercises and types of equipment. For the majority of your arm training, it's best to use free weights and slowly work your way into adding machine variations, such as cable curls and triceps pushdowns. Exercises including long bar curls, dumbbell curls, the close grip bench press, and triceps dips are all great mass builders.

By comparison, machine exercises such as cable curls and triceps rope pushdowns are more isolation movements, often referred to as "toning" exercises. Using exercise bands is also a very popular option. Because of the basic way a band works, more muscle is used as the band is stretched. These are great additions to your workout if you're working out at home or your gym has bands with handles. Bands are made to equal weights up to 100 pounds.

Arms are trained with both high reps with low weight and low reps with high weights. Keep reps in the 8–12 window when you start out because hypertrophy (muscle growth) occurs in this range. Making use of your 50–75 percent one rep max weight is the standard weight to follow for your reps. You'll want to build strength and endurance and strengthen your tendons and ligaments, but arms should not be trained hard in the first two months because of the extra work they'll get in back, chest, and shoulder workouts. Less is more and the allowance of rest time will allow the muscles to fully rebuild.

Arms will grow with compound exercises as well as isolation exercises, but compound should always take precedent in your training. What you don't want to do is work the arms so much that they stop growing or don't grow with the rest of your body. Many guys train the arms more frequently and yet aren't doing what the muscles need to develop. They repeatedly perform isolation exercises with all sorts of burnout sets and achieve a pump and muscle endurance but never the growth they seek.

Biceps and triceps don't have to be trained on the same day, and starting out, you don't have to train them together until you feel comfortable. Instead focus on the form and contraction of each exercise and keep reminding yourself that every single rep gets you one step closer to your ultimate goal.

Exercises for triceps include:
- Parallel bar dips
- Bench dips
- Close grip bench press
- Behind the head dumbbell extension
- Straight bar pushdowns
- Rope pushdowns

- Skull crushers

Exercises for biceps include:
- Seated or standing dumbbell curls
- Long bar curls
- EZ bar curls
- EZ bar reverse curls
- Hammer curls
- Chin-ups
- Concentration curls

Important safety notes:
- DON'T CURL IN THE SQUAT RACK. This is Gym Rule #1. Why is this even a thing? The reason is because there's a long bar in the squat rack and low racks in which to set it between sets. Most gyms have a vertical rack of shorter barbells that work well for long bar curls and you won't have to use the squat rack. The only time you can use the squat rack for curls is if the gym is empty or there are three or four other squat racks available and no one is waiting for you to finish.
- Another common mistake is lifting your elbows at the top half of the curl or flaring them out to help complete the curl. This is done to avoid using only the biceps and it lets the shoulder help out with the motion.
- When doing curls of any type, you don't need to bring the dumbbell or barbell all the way up to touch the front of the shoulder. Stop the rep about two inches from the front of the shoulder because the biceps has already hit peak contraction.
- The long bar and barbell curls are not compound exercises. Because only one joint is moving (the elbow), they are isolation exercises. With biceps, you may find that

barbells hurt your wrist because of the twist, especially when extra weight is added. You may instead prefer to use an EZ bar, as the bar is bent to allow for a natural wrist angle. You can hold it with your hands positioned close or wide to vary the stress on the biceps muscles.

- You'll want to train the brachialis, which is the top part of the forearm, through hammer curls and reverse curls. The brachialis is part of the extensor muscles, which are opposite the flexor muscles and used in any gripping movement.

- One mistake I see often during triceps pushdowns (straight bars or V-handles) is when the lifter wraps a thumb around the attachment, creating stress on the wrist. I also commonly see the wrist curling back at the bottom and top of the movement, which is a masked way of creating more range of motion. The wrist should stay locked in place during the entire movement to keep as much tension on the triceps as possible.

- When it comes to skull crushers, you may have to modify or do a French press with dumbbells instead. If you experience any pain during skull crushers, leave them out of your routine. Modifications include bringing the bar farther back behind the head and extending it out at an angle instead of right overhead, which puts direct strain on the elbow joint.

- Also, when doing reverse dips on a bench, keep your body close to the bench. Don't put plates on your thighs until you've been doing the exercise in your workouts for many months.

Biceps Workouts

Beginner
Seated dumbbell curls: 3 sets of 10
Standing dumbbell hammer curls: 3 sets of 10
EZ bar reverse curls: 3 sets of 10

Intermediate
Seated dumbbell curls: 4 sets of 8
Standing dumbbell hammer curls: 3 sets of 8
EZ bar reverse curls: 3 sets of 8

Intermediate-Advanced
Standing long bar curls: 4 sets of 10
Seated dumbbell curls: 4 sets of 10
Seated dumbbell hammer curls: 4 sets of 10
EZ bar reverse curls: 3 sets of 10

Advanced
Standing long bar curls: 4 sets of 8
Seated dumbbell hammer curls: 3 sets of 8
EZ bar reverse curls: 3 sets of 10
Rope hammer curls: failure
Cable curls: failure

Triceps Workouts

Beginner
Diamond push-ups: 3 sets of 10
Bench dips: 3 sets of 10
Behind the head dumbbell press: 3 sets of 10

Intermediate
Close grip bench press: 3 sets of 10
Parallel bar dips: 2 sets of 8
Bench dips: 3 sets of 10

Intermediate-Advanced
Close grip bench press: 3 sets of 8
Parallel bar dips: 3 sets of 8
Bench dips: 3 sets of 10
French press: 3 sets of 10

Advanced
Close grip bench press: 3 sets of 8
Parallel dips (add weight if needed): 3 sets of 8
Behind the head two-hand dumbbell press: 3 sets of 8
Rope pushdowns: 3 sets of 8
Diamond push-ups to failure: 2 sets

CHAPTER 22

HOW TO TRAIN YOUR LEGS AND CALVES

Legs are one of the most popular water cooler topics at any gym. You'll hear some people complain about their pain from a previous leg day, and others say they have legs planned that day and dread it. This is because the legs are unlike any other body part. It's almost impossible to do a leg workout without elevating your heart rate and breathing hard. The legs also have more muscle than any other part of the body, so the strain on the body in general is much higher.

You'll often hear it said that someone with a large upper body and small lower body must have skipped leg day, but this isn't always the case. I've seen guys in the gym squatting hundreds of pounds who have small legs. The legs, like other muscles, are subject to genetics as far as their growth and potential for growth. Though they will get stronger, they may not grow much even after up to a year of training.

Another aspect of leg training is that you can train them with higher intensity than other body parts. As you progress, you'll do sets of squats, step-ups, and lunges that will push you to your brink. You'll have sets that make you question if you'll be able to finish each rep and wonder if you should quit. You may even become addicted to the intense soreness and want to push yourself more and more so that you feel like you gave the workout all you have. You may want to ease into harder and harder workouts, but you also need to be able to walk the next day.

Leg Day Warm-up

Warming up for leg day requires more than just walking from your car to the gym. A proper warm-up gets more blood flowing and improves the range of motion you will need as you move into your first exercise.

My leg training warm-up consists of an elliptical or stair climber machine for five minutes. Some people prefer to walk on the treadmill, but I don't think this is enough to get the leg muscles warmed up properly. Early in your journey, the stair climber may be too much because your legs get tired a few minutes into it. If this is the case, do a couple of minutes on the stair machine after doing three to four minutes on the elliptical.

After the cardio warm-up, I'll do 20–25 leg swings side to side and 20–25 front to back. Next, I'll do a set of 10–15 lunges on each leg and then 25 bodyweight squats. I may add a few step-ups on the bench before my first exercise to get a little extra movement in the hips. After that, it's right into my first set of squats, starting with no weight and working my way up to my starting weight. As far as warm-ups go for any body part, you have to find what works best for you.

Leg and calf exercises include:
- Squats: barbell, goblet
- Step-ups
- Lunges: static, walking
- Glute/ham raises
- Leg presses
- Leg extension

- Standing calf raise
- Seated calf raise

Squats

No exercise requires more determination than the barbell squat. The feeling of loading up a weight on the bar and getting under it can either pump you up or make you uneasy. Every rep must be intentional and performed with a full range of motion. At the end of every set, you may have to convince yourself that you can do it again. But by your last set, you'll feel a strong sense of accomplishment and become addicted to the feeling. You may not love squats or leg day when you begin your journey but eventually, you'll look forward to them.

It's important to understand the mechanics of a proper squat. Don't add weight to the exercise in the form of dumbbells or a barbell until you observe correct form. Reading cues from a magazine and seeing photos of a proper squat may be enough for some of you, but for others, watching videos or observing a trainer at the gym will be more effective. Squatting correctly from the start will lead to long-term gains and help keep you injury free.

When squatting, go as low as you feel comfortable until you are eventually able to squat to parallel with the ground or slightly lower. You may hear people telling you not to go below parallel in the squat but this isn't necessarily true. The only reason some squat to parallel is that it's what the standard lifting competitions use as a gauge to judge whether a lift is complete.

Here are some important tips to ensure proper squat form:
- Always keep your knees lined up with your feet.
- Keep the knees in line with the ankles as much as possible as you descend into the squat. Don't let your knees push past your toes.
- Never adjust your feet mid-set.

- Be careful not to perform a "ballerina" lift off where you have to come up high on your toes to remove the bar from the squat rack. That means the bar is too high.
- You may need a pad across the bar when learning to squat, but as your traps and upper back muscles develop, you'll be able to more comfortably rest the bar directly on your back without the aid of the pad. If possible, make sure you have your workout buddy see if you are positioned in the dead center of the bar.
- Always keep a neutral spine (back not arched) throughout the lift, and don't look up from the bottom of the squat as you stand. Keep your gaze pointed forward to determine how low you are going.
- Don't allow gravity to do the lowering portion of the lift. Practice full control from top to bottom.
- Always brace the core and tighten the abs.
- Breathe in on the way down and breathe out on the way up.
- Don't let your ankles and knees cave in.
- Don't lift your heels off the ground.

I also recommend doing squats in a low-profile shoe without a lot of padding. The cushioning can compress during heavy squats and cause you to be unsteady. A lower profile shoe will help you feel more connected to the ground.

Also, don't do half reps for the majority of your reps. Make sure to go as low as you feel comfortable and return to a full standing position. If you need to do a half rep on the final rep because you can't finish it, that's okay.

Box squats

The box squat may be worth adding into your workouts, especially to help you work on your depth in the squat. The box squat is performed by setting a box at or slightly below the depth you usually squat. Instead of tapping the box, sit down on it fully without losing tension in your back, core, and lower body. The goal is to stop the movement fully and then come back up without using momentum.

Pause squats

The pause squat can be another excellent variation for breaking plateaus. It's done by going only to the bottom of the squat, maintaining good form, and pausing for a length of time making the squat much harder with your chosen weight.

Lunges

When lunging, keep the upper body upright to make your quads work more than the glutes. When you step back into a lunge, also try to keep weight on the front foot's heel to keep the knee from going over the toe.

Workouts

Beginner
Body weight squats: 3 sets of 15
Body weight back lunges: 3 sets of 12
Body weight step-ups: 3 sets of 10

Beginner-Intermediate
Goblet squats: 4 sets of 12
Back lunges: holding dumbbells at your side – 3 sets of 12
Step-ups: holding dumbbells at your side – 2 sets of 12

Intermediate
Barbell squats: 3 sets of 10
Barbell back lunges: 3 sets of 10
Glute raises: 3 sets of 10
Step-ups: 3 sets of 10

Intermediate-Advanced
Barbell squats: 4 sets of 10
Barbell back lunges: 4 sets of 8
Step-ups: 4 sets of 8
Glute raise: 4 sets of 10
Wall sit to failure: 3 sets

Advanced
Barbell squats: 3 sets of 8
Walking lunges: barbell or dumbbells at your side – 3 sets of 8
RDL: 3 sets of 8
Glute raise: 3 sets of 8
Leg extension: 3 sets of 10

Calf Training

The calves are essential for a balanced physique. Some men luck out and have bigger calves due to genetics. Their calf muscles stay well developed with daily activities, but for most men, this isn't the case. The calves are an area where almost everyone suffers aesthetically. It can be extremely challenging to add size, especially with someone who has naturally small or skinny calves. The calves are used throughout most of our day and are therefore adept at taking a high load. But to grow, they require a continual extra stimulus and an understanding of their muscle composition.

The calf has two components: The gastrocnemius and the soleus muscles. Two muscle heads comprise the gastrocnemius, and they run from slightly above the knee down to the heel and are located on the very back of the lower leg. It's made up mostly of fast twitch muscles, which respond to more weight and fewer reps to get them to grow. The gastrocnemius, or gastroc, is used primarily in running and jumping and less in walking. It's trained by exercises such as standing calf raises and leg press calf extensions.

The soleus, on the other hand, lies beneath the gastrocnemius and is mostly slow twitch fibers. It's primarily in use while standing and walking and also used in running to a lesser degree. It can be worked only during bent-knee exercises such as seated calf raises.

If it's your first session training the calves, or first few sessions, don't push them extra hard. You can tack a calf workout on to your leg day, but as you advance, it should be done on your off days from other muscles. On a scale of 1 to 10, your first calf workout should be a 2 or 3. Slowly work into training them, and after a few weeks, you can then push them as hard as you'd like.

If you work them too hard during that first workout, you won't be able to put much weight or stress on them for the next few days. Walking up and down stairs will be especially painful until the muscles can relax. They will feel excruciatingly tight and, with lots of stretching, will take about two to three days to relax completely. You could do a repeat of your first workout for the second session and they won't feel as tight as they did after that first workout. If you start working calves consistently for a few months or weeks and then drop off, you will more than likely feel this pain again next time you work them. My advice isn't to stop training them, no matter what.

If they're not growing after months of training, change up your routine by doing more weight and lower reps or more reps with less weight. For most men, three sets of standing calf raises at the end of a leg workout isn't enough to get them to grow. There are many ways to work the calves but you have to work them correctly and consistently. The form you use on any calf exercise can make or break your results.

As you get more comfortable with calf training, you can push past the top end range of motion during a standing or calf raise. This simply means squeezing at the top of the move and then raising up just a tiny bit more to activate a bit more muscle before lowering the heels. If your chosen weight doesn't allow for end range of motion at the top, lower it by 5 pounds and try again.

Gastrocnemius training

Before starting your calf training, I recommend warming them up on a Stairmaster to increase blood flow and prepare the joints. If this isn't available, you can do 25–50 body weight standing calf raises after walking on the treadmill for four to five minutes. I also suggest you train your calves in a shoe that has very little cushion. This allows for more range of motion and more direct contact with your training surface.

Standing Calf Raises

One of the best methods to work the gastrocnemius are standing calf raises in the Smith machine. You will need to stand on some type of block that is at least two inches off the ground. Many gyms have a calf raise block stored near the Smith machines. This block is typically very stable and has grip tape on top so your toes don't slip during the calf raise. If you train at home and don't have one, they can be purchased online, or some people construct their own out of two-by-fours. If the gym doesn't have a calf raise block, you can use the edge of flat plates from 25 pounds and up, laid on the ground. Simply position the block or plates directly under the Smith machine bar, making sure your toes and feet are not angled behind or in front of you. They need to be directly underneath you.

For a standing calf raise, place your feet about shoulder-width apart keeping the knees ever so slightly bent. You want to position the Smith machine bar across the upper back standing as tall as possible. I prefer to use a squat pad on the bar to keep the bar from digging into my traps and upper back. The balls of your feet should be dead center on the edge of the object you are standing on, allowing your heels plenty of room to drop.

Your focus should be on the big toe to help target the outer the part of the gastrocnemius or outer toes for the inner. You can't completely isolate each area but it helps to define it. Also, don't twist your feet during calf raises, in or out. You can distribute the weight across all of the toes to work the calf overall.

You'll often see people at the gym incorrectly doing bouncing calf raises and this is usually combined with a short range of motion. In calf training, there is a debate about whether to drop the heels all the way to the ground or to stop when the foot is flat. My suggestion is to drop the heels down and feel the stretch at the bottom. In between calf sets, you can stretch the calf muscle by placing the foot up on a step and angling it slightly inward while pressing the heel towards the ground. Since the fascia around the calf can limit calf growth, it's good to stretch it.

Leg Press Calf Raises

Another popular method of training the gastrocnemius is to lie back on a leg press with the balls of your feet on the bottom edge of the push platform. Keeping the legs almost completely straight, drop the heels down and then press the foot up to move the platform up a couple inches. Squeeze at the top of the motion and then come down slow. I'd start out with just the weight of the platform, or sled, before adding weight.

You can also stand on a calf raise block while wearing a weight vest, or holding a dumbbell in one hand, making sure you grip something with the free hand for balance.

Soleus training

Solcus training is done differently than gastroc training. While the gastroc is worked standing up with the leg almost totally straightened, the soleus is worked by seated training. The seated calf raise machine is common in bigger gyms. If one isn't available, I'll give you instructions on how to set up the Smith machine to double as one.

Seated Calf Raise

The seated calf raise machine is a seat with two foot holds in front of it, knee pads underneath, and a bar that holds weight plates on each side. To use it, load up your starting weight. I suggest one 10-pound weight on each side if it's your first time training calves. Next, place your feet on the foot holds and then slide the top bar down and press it as tightly as possible on top of your knees. The ball of your foot should be on the back edge of the foot holds, allowing your heel to drop down. I have found the best rep count for doing seated calf raises is two seconds up, pause and squeeze at the top, and one second down with a one-second pause at the bottom. Be sure not to bounce, especially when trying to squeeze out the last few reps.

If you don't have access to a seated calf raise machine, you can use a Smith machine. To begin, bring the bar down until it's about three feet off the ground. Next, slide the end of a flat bench up in front of the bar. You'll be sitting on the end of the bench with your knees under the bar. Your calves should be under you in a 90-degree position with your feet resting on a calf raise block or another object. Use a pad across the bar so it doesn't dig into your thighs. Un-rack the Smith machine bar by twisting it and lifting slightly so all of the weight is resting on your knees. Maintain the same rep count and motion as when you use a seated calf raise machine.

Workouts

Beginner
Smith machine standing calf raise: 4 sets of 15
Seated calf raise: 3 sets of 15
Body weight calf raise: 1 set of 25 slow

Intermediate
Smith machine standing calf raise: 4 sets of 15

Seated calf raise: 4 sets of 12
Body weight calf raise: 1 set of 50 slow

Intermediate-Advanced
Smith machine standing calf raise: 5 sets of 10
Seated calf raise: 3 sets of 15
Body weight calf raise: 3 sets of 25 slow

Advanced
Smith machine standing calf raise: 4 sets of 20
Seated calf raise: 3 sets of 10
Standing bodyweight calf raise: 3 sets to failure

CHAPTER 23

HOW TO TRAIN YOUR ABS

The abs are one area that almost everyone trains hard but they don't always see the results they want. For starters, you will need less than 9 percent body fat to reveal the abs, otherwise you can't see the muscles. I've seen many people who are more than 20–50 pounds overweight doing ab machines in hopes of having the coveted six pack. But without proper nutrition, no amount of crunches will ever change how your stomach looks.

You may not know the difference between the core and the abs. The core applies to your abdominals, obliques, and low back muscles, all of which are important to train. The lower back is typically undertrained, and if you are doing only crunching motions, you will start to feel lower back tension and sometimes pain until it's properly developed. Having a strong core is extremely important to protect the lower back during certain exercises and to assist with daily activities such as picking up a bag of mulch or a heavy box.

You can do abs every other day, but if you are just starting out, you may want to do them twice a week in case your stomach muscles and lower back become too sore after the workout. If you are looking to purchase ab training equipment at home, you can purchase a stability ball or a heavily padded mat to provide cushioning for your elbows and back. Regardless of the ab exercise, make sure you contract the muscles and keep them engaged.

Here is a basic ab routine that you can modify to make easier or more challenging by increasing/decreasing reps or time:

Beginner
Bird dogs (not alternating): 1 sets of 10
Crunches: 1 sets of 10
Planks: 1 sets for 30 seconds
Supermans: 1 sets of 10

Intermediate
Bird dogs (not alternating): 2 sets of 10
Crunches: 3 sets of 10
Planks: 2 sets for 30 seconds
Supermans: 1 set of 10

Advanced
Captain's chair knees hold: 3 sets of 30 seconds
Captain's chair (knee raises, starting with knees at 90 degrees, and then bringing them to chest): 3 sets of 10

Do each exercise slowly and make each rep burn as much as possible.

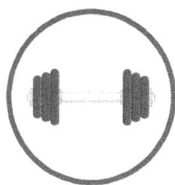

PART 5:
ONWARD!

CHAPTER 24

ADDITIONAL TRAINING

Fitness classes can help you stay on track and provide additional fitness benefits. They come in all shapes and sizes from spin and group training to full-body barbell classes and everything in between. The class environment can be a great motivator if you are feeling lazy or want something different to add to your training. Excellent for conditioning, classes also can give you a new training stimulus. Many gyms offer classes free with membership, but others may charge per class or have monthly rates. Instructors lead classes, which means you don't have to worry about putting together a workout.

A good starting choice is a full-body barbell class where you decide how much weight to add to the bar. Be conservative here. If you load up the bar with two 10-pound plates on each side, you'll find very quickly that you may not be able to finish the class. You'll have to stop and reduce the weight while everyone stares at you or you risk being called out by the instructor. These classes will work the entire body with exercises such as curls, lunge combos, squats, and press combos. Not only are they challenging but you'll be doing exercises you don't normally do with a different rep count or time than usual.

Some gyms may have classes focusing on a specific piece of equipment, such as TRX or kettlebell. Though you may feel uncomfortable in your first class, keep going and you'll soon find yourself upset if you miss the class. Some classes have three or four instructors who teach at different times, and many people will schedule the class specifically because of the instructor. Some classes are motivating while others focus on your desired goals.

Ab classes are also available at certain gyms and usually full of people expecting to get six-pack results in a week. However, the abs can be seen only if body fat is low enough. If you decide to take one of these classes, remember that it's to work your core and not lose fat.

Yoga classes are very popular and now offered by most gyms as well as yoga studios. I highly recommend doing yoga even once a week for the many benefits it offers, such as increased balance and flexibility as well as tapping into your breathing. Start out with the easiest class and work your way up.

CHAPTER 25

MEASURING YOUR PROGRESS

Taking your measurements each month can be exciting, especially at the end of a month where you can see visible increases. Compare your measurements and weight logs with the previous month, as well as your starting measurements, to see how far you've come. The changes can be eye-opening.

With photos, I always like adding a filter on my phone to make them black and white, which highlights muscle definition. You can print out pictures and keep them in a binder for doing a side-by-side comparison or you can view them on a computer.

You'll make your most significant gains during the first year of training. The longer you train, the more effort it will take to keep improving your gains due to the law of diminishing returns. You'll notice this as your growth and strength begins to decrease, even as you lift more and heavier weights.

It can also be important to reevaluate your nutrition. At the end of each month, make sure you are adding enough calories if you are increasing intensity and volume. If you begin to see a plateau, I'd suggest adding an entirely different type of workout, such as a strength-style workout class that involves more cardio. You can also try adding a day of using bodyweight exercises with higher reps. Doing this will give your body an entirely different stimulus and can even break up the monotony of day-to day-weights.

CHAPTER 26
CARDIO CLIMBING

The goal of this book is to teach you how to build muscles, but there is one muscle we have not covered yet: The heart. The heart is strengthened through various forms of cardio. Cardio, or cardiovascular training, is aerobic exercise from low to high intensity that requires oxygen for its energy demands.

Along with improving heart functioning, cardiovascular endurance is important for many aspects of life. You'll need it if you want to be able to take three flights of stairs without getting out of breath or complete a long hike with your family and not fall behind. You'll work your cardiovascular system during leg exercises as well as certain upper body exercises, like pull-ups and push-ups, and it needs to be able to keep up with your workouts.

Your heart also needs to be strong to support your body's accumulation of muscle mass, and your body type will determine how much cardio you should be doing. If you are someone who has difficulty building muscle and is very lean, you will need to limit the amount of cardio because too much can impact your muscle gains. I suggest two days of low-intensity cardio per week, such as walking or elliptical at a pace that keeps your heart rate between 60–65 percent.

If you are someone with high body fat and are naturally larger, you will want to mix steady state cardio such as treadmill walking with one to two days of high intensity interval training to burn the fat, expose the muscle, and improve cardio.

If you have a high metabolism and an easier ability to add muscle, your cardio range can be less. One to two days of high intensity intervals won't affect your gains.

High intensity interval training (HIIT) is simply performing an exercise for a short burst of time, resting for a set period, and returning to the exercise for 10 rounds or a set time limit. An example of common HIIT is walking for 30 seconds and then running for 15 seconds, doing each back and forth for a max of 20 minutes total. Another is performing burpees in the same 30 seconds on, 30 seconds off format.

Burpees are accomplished by placing your hands on the floor or a bench in a push-up position. Hop your feet close to your upper body, jump in the air, and then jump your feet out to the starting push-up position. This type of cardio burns a lot of calories and keeps your body in a fat burning state for hours after the workout. That's due to an effect called Exercise Post Oxygen Consumption (EPOC). Instead of naturally burning one to two calories, the body burns anywhere from four to six calories per minute at rest.

Can you perform cardio while trying to build muscle? The short answer is, yes. Cardio should be done doing workouts that also build muscle—for instance, riding a bike, using battle ropes, or swimming. If you're worried about your heart rate getting too high, you can do steady state cardio such as walking or using an elliptical, keeping the heart rate in the 60–65 percent range where the body taps into fat for its sole energy source.

Cardio between workouts, on your off days, also can help with muscle recovery. For example, you could do a light bike ride the day after doing a leg workout. Swimming is also a great recovery cardio option.

The best time for cardio differs from person to person. The best time is going to be the time that works consistently week after week for you. I don't recommend doing a cardio session before your weight training workouts, however. Save it for your day off, and your lighter cardio can be done during a rest day.

CHAPTER 27

REACHING THE SUMMIT

Continuing to train hard and strain your body during each workout can take a toll in the form of muscle knots, tightness, and overall fatigue. It's vital that you keep your body performing optimally between your sessions. The first requirement, and most vital, is ensuring you get enough sleep.

Sleep

Your muscles repair and grow while you sleep, not when you train. If you're staying up late and waking up early every day, lack of sleep isn't only going to affect your workouts but also your growth. I suggest getting to bed at the same time each night if possible, especially if you have to wake up early. Aim for at least six hours of sleep a night, adding an hour or two if you still don't feel rested.

Staring at your phone or a computer screen can impact your ability to fall asleep, so I suggest putting away devices at least an hour before your intended bedtime. You can also try drinking a calming herbal tea or reading a book if that helps you feel drowsy. If you finish training and then head home to get to bed, your body may be energized making sleep extra difficult to achieve. If this is the case, you may need to adjust your training time.

Also, be sure not to have caffeine at least 8–10 hours before bed. I don't recommend using a caffeinated pre-workout after 1:00 p.m. If possible, you can take a 20-minute power nap in your afternoon if it gives you the energy you need to hit your evening workout.

Massage

The second way to make sure your body is in top form is to get frequent massages. If you've never had a massage, or have any preconceptions about them, I suggest you try one to see the positive effects it has on your body. Finding a good massage therapist can take some time, and I suggest finding someone who has a private practice. I suggest trying a male and a female massage therapist to see which you prefer.

The most common massages are Swedish and deep tissue, and you can try both to see which one you like best. A deep tissue massage allows the therapist to really work the muscles and release any knots, which will leave your body feeling less restricted in its range of motion during your next workout. Swedish, on the other hand, leads to more overall releasing of the muscles without terribly deep pressure. Both types of massages also help encourage blood flow, which also benefits your entire body. I suggest getting a massage at least once a month but bimonthly is okay too.

CHAPTER 28

PERSONAL TRAINERS

Sometimes it makes sense to hire a personal trainer to help demonstrate exercises and keep you accountable. There are a lot of very good trainers out there but others are just rep counters and don't have your best interest or a plan in mind. By following the recommendations in this chapter, you'll know from the very first meeting whether or not a trainer is the right fit for you.

Many big box gyms provide personal trainers and will even offer free sessions to get you started. Most trainers will show you around the gym, explain how to properly use the equipment, and provide fitness testing at your first session. Use caution; the purpose of free training sessions is often for the trainer to sell you a package.

First and foremost, you want to find a trainer who fits with your training goals. One option is to observe trainers at your current gym working out on their own to see if they train themselves the way you want to be trained. Their physiques will show if they practice what they preach.

Another good way to find the right trainer is to speak to the gym's fitness director or whoever supervises trainers at your gym. You can discuss your training goals and your desired training style.

You can also search online for trainers in your area at boutique personal training studios and read their reviews. A personal training studio can provide a more private experience.

If you have any type of injury, tell your trainer before you sign up with them. Be absolutely sure that they're able to work around it and still provide results. You may have to remind them of your issue during the first few sessions or let them know that you are unable to perform a specific exercise or angle. If they tell you to work around it and don't modify the exercise, it's time to find another trainer.

After you sign up, be sure to discuss your goals in detail and ensure that they're SMART goals. This acronym stands for Specific, Measurable, Attainable, Relevant, and Timely. The trainer should have both a short- and long-term plan from the first session and not just give you randomized workouts. Also, make sure they provide a proper initial assessment of your current fitness level and take all of your measurements as well as a photo.

When it comes to your workouts as a whole, you can use your trainer as a complete guide to your journey, or you can have them take you progressively through one or all of the routines in this book. The number of days a week you train with them will determine the split they give you. You can also tell them that you would like only a conditioning-style workout, which is strength combined with cardio for full body fitness.

A trainer can also be used to check your form on exercises if you want to do your own routine. You can arrange to meet them once a week to help you through a certain workout if you are uncertain of how to safely perform it.

There are many benefits to having a personal trainer. For starters, with a trainer showing you the correct form for exercises, you will be less likely to be injured, which could possibly set your progress back weeks or even months. You'll also move forward much faster by being pointed in the right direction for relevant exercises and routines, which removes the element of guessing at workouts and making minimal gains.

A trainer also provides accountability for those days when you don't want to work out or are lacking motivation. Knowing that someone you've paid is waiting for you can be enough to get you off the couch or out of bed and to your workout. A good trainer will also provide constant motivation and enthusiasm throughout your workout.

Even if you have been training for a while, hiring a trainer can help you break through a plateau or introduce you to new exercises, especially for a body part you don't enjoy training. Hiring someone for a workout you don't enjoy can make it less agonizing.

A good trainer won't give you a diet but may offer nutritional advice. Unless they also happen to be a dietitian, it's out of their scope of practice to give you a meal plan. They can suggest different options for snacks and meals but can't give exact portion sizes or lay out an entire plan.

Finding the right trainer will have a big impact on your overall results and enjoyment of your workouts. Some people like having a trainer who talks a lot while others prefer someone who is quieter, pushing them hard enough to where there is no time to talk. The trainer's personality, training style, and overall look are important factors to look for a match.

Check your area for prices and if you're on a budget, consider shorter 30-minute sessions. Some gyms also offer discounts for six month or annual commitments, saving you on cost per session.

Working out with an at-home personal trainer, even once a month, can be a great option if you have the proper equipment. Some trainers can bring some smaller equipment with them, but this typically consists of a few dumbbells, an exercise ball, and some bands. A good trainer can adapt the workout to the equipment and give you a great workout. They also should be giving you workouts to do on your own and a way to track your progress.

My hope is that you will be able to achieve your desired look without having to hire a personal trainer, though they may be an asset when you get started.

CHAPTER 29

THE ROAD AHEAD

I wrote this book in the hopes of improving the lives and bodies of many people. My sincerest wish is that you find great value in the guidance it provides. I also hope that it gives you the motivation to get in shape if you've been putting it off. This journey never ends, and you can do something every day to improve and tune your physique or make it stronger.

Though the trail ahead may seem like an uphill climb, keep going and always look back to see how far you've traveled, not how far you have left to go.

Best of luck, and see you on the trail!

Jeremy

Acknowledgements

I want to give a thank you to everyone who helped me along the way with the writing of this book and special thanks for Maurice Browne and Elizabeth Phillips.

www.ingramcontent.com/pod-product-compliance
Lightning Source LLC
Chambersburg PA
CBHW060336030426
42336CB00011B/1376